P9-ELW-263

THE JUICE GENERATION

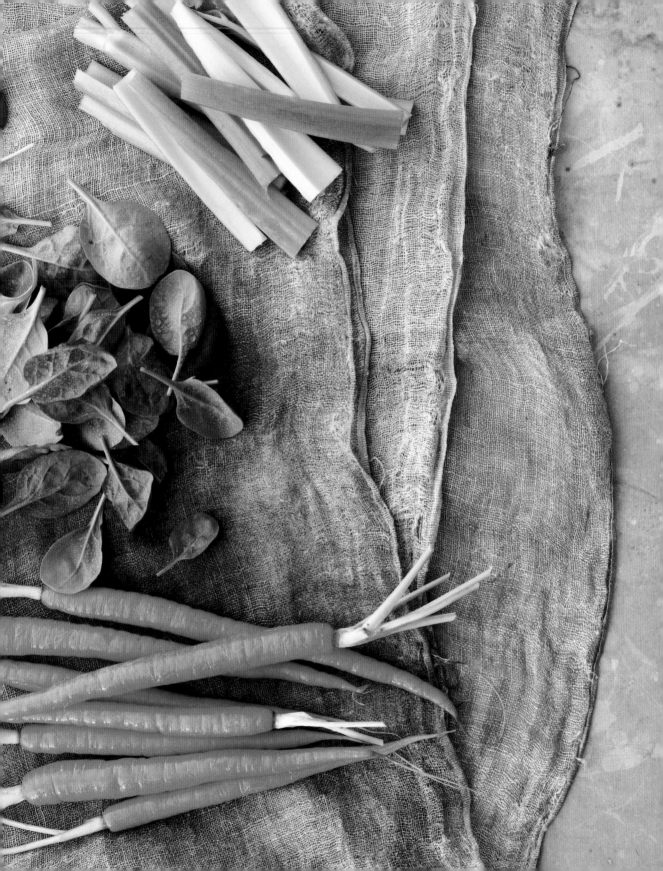

THE JUICE GENERATION

100 RECIPES FOR FRESH JUICES AND SUPERFOOD SMOOTHIES

ERIC HELMS

with Amely Greeven

Marc Balet
Creative Director

Foreword by
Salma Hayek

A Touchstone Book

Published by Simon & Schuster
New York   London   Toronto   Sydney   New Delhi

Who Should Use Caution When Juicing and Blending:

You should consult with your doctor before starting a cleanse program and we advocate caution for some, including:

- Women who are pregnant or breast-feeding should check with their health provider about juicing. It's wiser to wait until after breast-feeding to indulge in the ultra-detox-promoting ingredients mentioned in Phase 3.
- Anyone with a weakened immune system (the elderly, the very young, and those on chemotherapy treatment) should purchase only the freshest produce, and take extra care when washing. Be sure to discuss juicing with their health provider to ensure safe cleansing.
- People with diabetes or hypoglycemia, and those who know they have candida (yeast overgrowth in the intestines) should learn the right way to juice for their bodies and are strongly advised to get guidance from a health provider on a healthy, low-sugar juicing habit.
- Anyone who is using medication should always consult his or her health provider about possible food contraindications.

The Juice Generation
100 Recipes for Fresh Juices and Superfood Smoothies
Eric Helms
with Amely Greeven

Touchstone
A Division of Simon & Schuster, Inc.
1230 Avenue of the Americas
New York, NY 10020

Copyright © 2014 by Eric Helms, LLC.
Design: Tyler Mintz/Cristina Vásquez Obando

Still Life photography: © William Brinson
Lifestyle photography: © John Huba

JUICE GENERATION and Design®, HAIL TO KALE®, SUPA DUPA GREENS®, VITAL SHOT®, and PROTEIN BUZZ® are registered service marks, and JUICE GENERATION℠, PEANUT BUTTER SPLIT℠, PB ACAI℠, LEMON LOZENGE℠, COCO ACAI℠, JUICE FARMACY℠, and COLD WARRIOR℠ are common law service marks, of Juice Generation, Inc.

All rights reserved, including the right to reproduce this book or portions thereof in any form whatsoever. For information address Touchstone Subsidiary Rights Department, 1230 Avenue of the Americas, New York, NY 10020.

This publication contains the opinions and ideas of its author. It is intended to provide helpful and informative material on the subjects addressed in the publication. It is sold with the understanding that the author and publisher are not engaged in rendering medical, health, or any other kind of personal professional services in the book. The reader should consult his or her medical, health or other competent professional before adopting any of the suggestions in this book or drawing inferences from it.

The author and publisher specifically disclaim all responsibility for any liability, loss or risk, personal or otherwise, which is incurred as a consequence, directly or indirectly, of the use and application of any of the contents of this book.

First Touchstone trade paperback edition January 2014

TOUCHSTONE and colophon are registered trademarks of Simon & Schuster, Inc.

For information about special discounts for bulk purchases, please contact Simon & Schuster Special Sales at 1-866-506-1949 or business@simonandschuster.com.

The Simon & Schuster Speakers Bureau can bring authors to your live event. For more information or to book an event contact the Simon & Schuster Speakers Bureau at 1-866-248-3049 or visit our website at www.simonspeakers.com.

Manufactured in the United States of America

5 7 9 10 8 6 4

ISBN 978-1-4767-4568-8
ISBN 978-1-4767-4570-1 (ebook)

7

FOREWORD

by Salma Hayek

10

WELCOME TO THE JUICE GENERATION!

44

THE GREEN CURVE

72

PHASE 1: Light Green:

Bright and Refreshing

130

PHASE 2: Medium Green:

Take Your Juice to the Next Level

174

PHASE 3: Ultra Green:

The Full Feel-Good Effect

212

CLEANSE AND REVIVE

Using Your Juicing Tools for Detoxing and Healing

240

ABOUT THE AUTHOR

ACKNOWLEDGMENTS

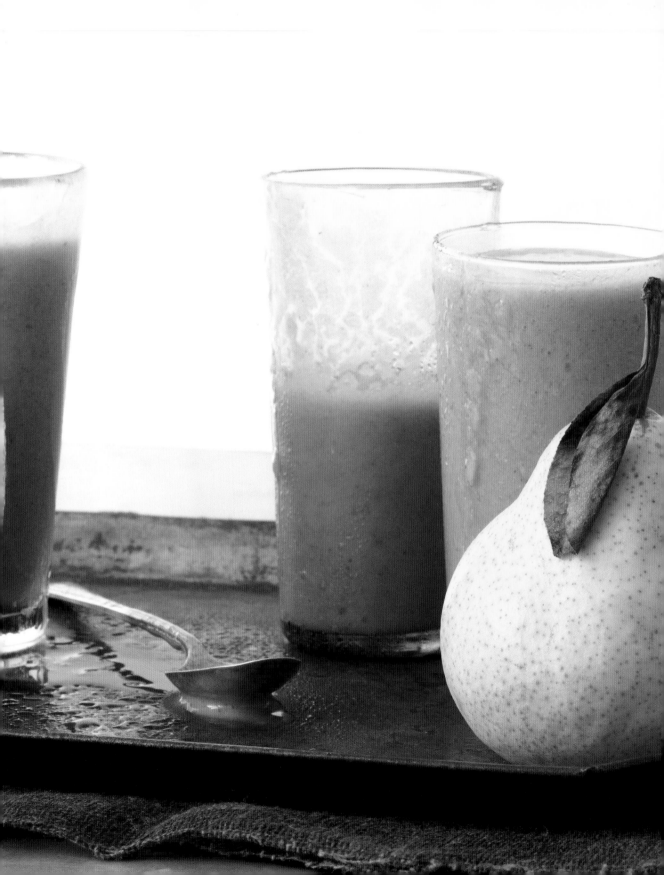

= FOREWORD =

Growing up in Coatzacoalcos, Veracruz, Mexico, aguas frescas—cooling drinks made of watermelon, cucumber, lime, *guanabana*, melon, prickly pear, tamarind, rice-based horchatas, hibiscus flower teas, to name a few—were always on the menu, instead of the traditional sodas. Savoring the colors, aromas, and tastes of these fresh-made juices was something I embraced at an early age.

When I moved to California in my midtwenties, I discovered a whole new world of juicing, one devoted to the healing effects of green juices squeezed from buckets of vegetables and tart citrus fruits. Green juicing was still something of a West Coast phenomenon at that time—mainly done by dedicated health nuts—and not nearly as accessible as it is today. But for me, it was love at first sip.

I started buying armfuls of California-grown cucumbers, celery, spinach, lemons, and grapefruits, and my kitchen—always my favorite room in my home—became my laboratory of liquid experiments. I loved the energy, the clarity in body and mind, and the glowing skin that my glasses of liquid green delivered. And, since I do find good meals to be a true source of pleasure—I believe eating well, and with people you love, is about feeding your body, heart, and soul—I used juicing to ensure I covered my nutritional bases every day, and as a tool to restore inner balance if my body needed a break from too much indulgence. I was one of the first people in my circle of friends to do short juice cleanses when I felt the need to get calm, clear, and focused and to give my body a chance to rest and restore. At the beginning, they looked at me a little strangely, but when they saw the results they understood that my homemade juices were key to my preventive healthcare regime: a way to keep equilibrium, take charge of my health, and look my very best.

That's always been what juicing is to me: a tool for staying in balance. Juicing vegetables and fruits, or drinking green smoothies, is not about deprivation or dieting. These are habits that help us add more to our lives: more high-grade, nutrition-rich foods in a busy, fast-paced schedule; more awareness of what our body needs to stay well and not get sick; and perhaps most important, more sensory delight from delicious foods that we otherwise might not try.

They're also life changing. Anyone who has, at the very least, a cheap blender, can begin to drink their way to well-being by tripling or quadrupling their daily dose of fresh vegetables and fruits in about three minutes. This has wonderful effects for everyone, no matter where on the eating spectrum they are. To me, this is what the current juice boom is all about: people of all ages discovering their power to feel and look better by giving their bodies the essential elements they need.

As a mother, I have even more reason to get fruits and vegetables into the juicer. I want my daughter to grow up learning to love all the benefits that nature offers. I am also happy that proceeds from this book are going to Wellness in the Schools, a pioneering nonprofit program that brings chefs and restaurateurs into New York City's public school cafeterias and classrooms, alongside fitness and environmental experts, to combat childhood obesity and give every kid a chance to be their best and brightest self.

When I met Eric Helms fifteen years ago, it was like finding a juicing coconspirator—one who had access to the newest, coolest ingredients on the natural-foods scene. Eventually, we launched a juice-cleanse delivery service using the recipes we'd developed. We called it Cooler Cleanse, and our mission was to give busy people a simple way to recharge and renew themselves, using cold-pressed juices and raw-food meals in moderate cleansing and detox programs.

Eric's book, *The Juice Generation*, is driven by the same mission of making juicing and blending accessible, exciting, and even more important, a long-term, "happy green habit" that doesn't get dropped after a two-week fling. It confronts the myth that things that are great for us don't always taste good. With its three-phase program of recipes, this book offers an innovative solution; a culinary adventure that tempts you into the world of green and nutrient-dense drinks slowly and deliciously, one step at a time, so your taste buds can adjust from sweet to savory naturally. It could convert anyone from juice skeptic to juice connoisseur!

Juicing and blending help me stay energized and positive, and bring me back to center if I wander a little too far into the tempting pleasures of wine, pasta, and cheese. I hope that you and those you love will enjoy the adventure of drinking your food as much as I have—and that this book gives you the skills and inspiration to make your own kitchen an exciting, colorful, liquid laboratory, too.

Salma Hayek

WELCOME TO THE JUICE GENERATION!

Do you live juicy? Are you energized and uplifted, with a little extra spring in your step? Does your skin glow? Do your eyes shine? Is your mind clear and your outlook optimistic? Do you feel light and bright inside?

If you answer yes, chances are that you're already a convert to the power of juicing and blending, got a green drink habit going on, and maybe even have a thing for superfood smoothies. The recipes in this book will expand your juice know-how with new flavors and combinations to explore.

But if your life is not as juicy as you'd like it to be, if you find yourself chasing the next latte, cola, or energy drink high, or you feel foggy or dull, get ready to experience the boost you can get from juice in all its splendid forms.

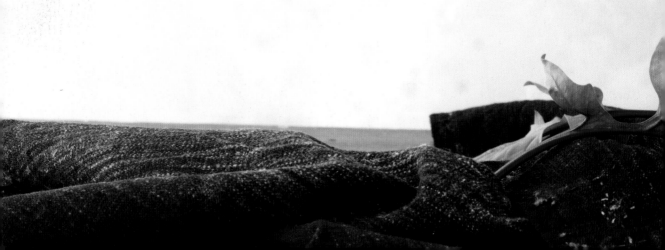

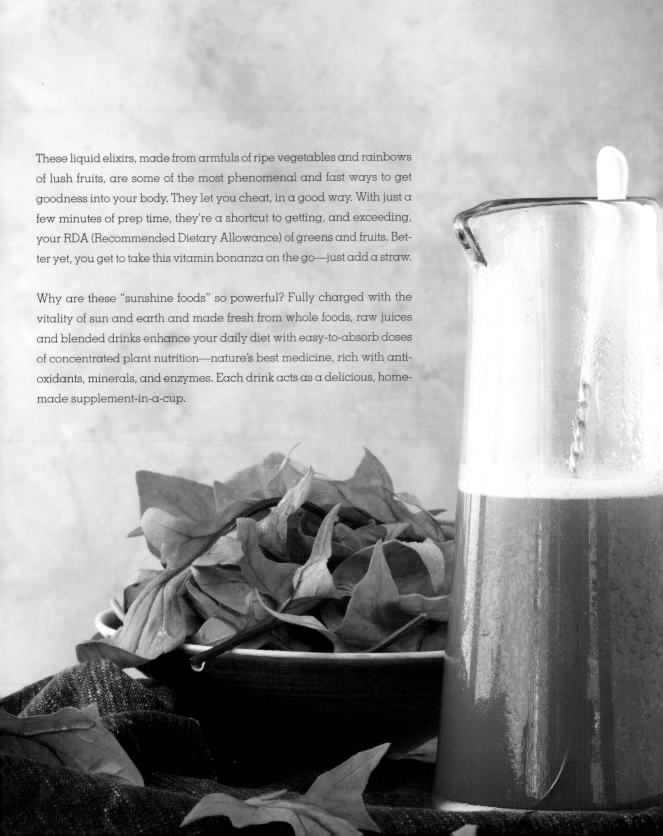

These liquid elixirs, made from armfuls of ripe vegetables and rainbows of lush fruits, are some of the most phenomenal and fast ways to get goodness into your body. They let you cheat, in a good way. With just a few minutes of prep time, they're a shortcut to getting, and exceeding, your RDA (Recommended Dietary Allowance) of greens and fruits. Better yet, you get to take this vitamin bonanza on the go—just add a straw.

Why are these "sunshine foods" so powerful? Fully charged with the vitality of sun and earth and made fresh from whole foods, raw juices and blended drinks enhance your daily diet with easy-to-absorb doses of concentrated plant nutrition—nature's best medicine, rich with antioxidants, minerals, and enzymes. Each drink acts as a delicious, homemade supplement-in-a-cup.

How much of your diet can you say that about? They protect your system against the stress and toxicity you face every day and they're potent antidotes to the fatiguing effects of a time-challenged, fast-paced modern life.

Juices also help you look fantastic. Famed for their rejuvenating properties, they give your skin a vibrant, healthy glow, help your eyes shine bright, help you maintain an ideal weight, and generally contribute to a younger and more vital appearance. And juices and smoothies fit into any dietary regimen with a caloric spectrum that runs from a supremely low 60 calories per 8 ounces of green juice; to a vitamin-stacked 120 calories for a slightly sweet 12-ounce fruit juice; to a rich and filling 400-calorie smoothie plumped with healthy fats. One swig of an emerald-green fruit-and-veggie nectar and you feel it instantly: You're revitalized, inspired, and poised for action.

Now we're inviting you to join the Juice Generation, to learn what making your own plant-filled concoctions can do for you, and for your family and friends. Whether you're a juice virgin, newly juice curious, or already an old pro with the single-auger juicer, we want to get you excited about the endless possibilities of squeezing, crushing, and grinding, and get you skilled in integrating the joys of juicing into your busy life.

For too long, a daily juicing habit has seemed out of reach—a complicated luxury that only devout yogis and the charmed elite manage to pull off. But the tide is changing, and now it's easier and more accessible than ever to integrate a short (and yes that can mean five-minute) juicing or blending ritual into your life. Incorporating these power foods does not require a whole lifestyle change: it's about picking up a few new tools and making this a happy habit—something that fits into the way you already live.

With a little guidance, some practice, and a willingness to try something new, you too can boost your body, mind, and spirit with nutrient-rich cocktails. The door is open—come on in!

JUICE GENERATION, THE STORE

Fifteen years ago, we started a small juice bar called, appropriately, Juice Generation, in the heart of—some would say the belly of—New York City, in Hell's Kitchen. It was a ballsy move: Back then, people would walk into our oxygenated oasis, look quizzically at our steel juicers, ask, "Where's the food?" and walk out. Public awareness of juicing was still a seed waiting to sprout.

But we persisted, making juices and smoothies fresh-to-order for a small band of loyal customers, because we sensed that the world's busiest city had a deep thirst for fresh-squeezed nourishment on-the-go. Our first fans were Broadway's hard-working actors and dancers, who relied on our juices and blended drinks to sustain them for long hours in rehearsal and on stage. They loved the light and clarifying refreshment they got from green juices and the heartier replenishment of recovery smoothies.

———

As foot traffic increased, we began to serve a bigger cross-section of Manhattanites, from harried professionals and fitness instructors, to toddler-toting moms. Our grassroots education in making liquid foods was earned from the best vantage point possible: behind a counter with a juicer and blender at the ready. Over the years, we've become pretty good at tempting people to take a walk on the raw side through juices and smoothies. We consider these drinks the ultraeasy, liquid aspect of the growing raw-food movement that is inspiring people to try out dishes made from "living" food like fresh greens and sprouted seeds and nuts. (They're just as delicious as a kelp-noodle pad thai or cashew coconut pie, and a lot less intimidating to make!) We also developed creative methods for helping people achieve smart and balanced juicing habits for the long term, like a "scale-up-the-green" ladder of drinks that helps beginners (who typically like sweeter things) introduce the all-important green vegetables into their cups slowly, so that their palates can adjust to the taste. We became international superfruit sleuths, adding yet undiscovered delicacies like pitaya (aka dragonfruit) to our recipes, because we were so excited about their nutritional potential and their unexpected flavor profiles. We even launched a sister company, Cooler Cleanse, offering detoxifying juice cleanses delivered to your door.

At Juice Generation, the store, our ethos is centered on making everything not just healthy but tasty. To us, enjoyment is part of well-being. If you consume healthy foods simply out of principle, and not out of pleasure, something's missing from the equation. You either lose the enthusiasm and drop the habit, or you keep going, but with a feeling of constriction or resentment—a state that is the opposite of vibrant health. Plus, we were motivated by sheer survival. Our Big Apple audience is filled with some of the world's most discerning foodies—chefs, restaurant critics, and the everyday patrons of the city's extraordinary food scene.

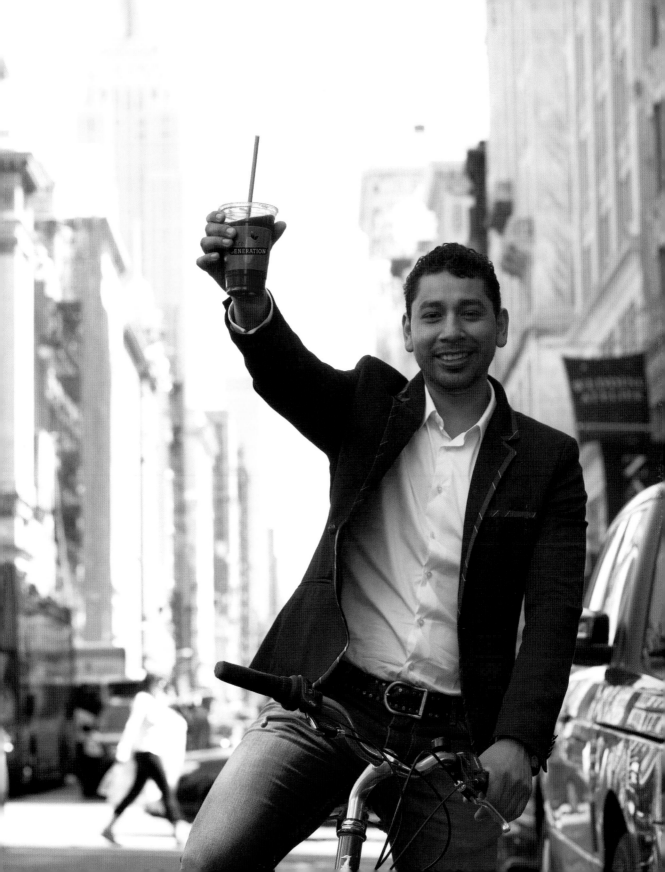

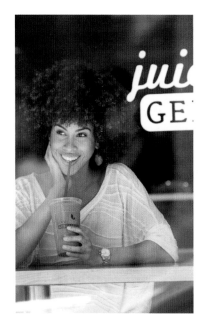

Our business has grown significantly since those pioneering Hell's Kitchen days, and now we're witnessing a juice boom in full swing. New York City is hopping with new juice bars, plant-based restaurants, and the latest iteration of this phenomenon: roaming juice trucks that bring their tonics straight to your street. Nationally, juice bars and juice cleansing companies are showing up in surprising pockets of America, and the exotic, food-as-medicine ingredients known as superfoods are filling the shelves in towns that previously had few natural-food options. The movement is taking off internationally, too, and the world of raw food and drink evolves daily online, with aficionados sharing daring new ingredients and exciting recipes that mix savory, sweet, spicy, and tangy with gusto.

Whether you're vegetarian or carnivore; a late-night pizza-eater or a Paleo-perfect fitness buff, getting daily doses of vegetables, fruits, nuts, seeds, sprouts, and superfoods in your drinks improves how you work, play, and live. And that's something to lift up your glass and toast.

I eat a lot at my restaurant, Telepan, and juicing is a way to get a good amount of nutrients into myself before I go in, without filling me up with calories. I've made it part of my daily routine, either by picking up a green juice on my way to work or making juice at home. And it is a great activity to do with the kids I work with at Wellness in the Schools (WITS)—it is a creative way to introduce them to fruit and vegetable combinations they might never have considered before.

—**Bill Telepan, celebrated chef; executive chef, Wellness in the Schools**

THE GREEN CURVE

We created this book to distill our fifteen years of wisdom into a field guide you can use to help you find juicing confidence in your own kitchen. We've created what we hope is a foolproof method that takes anyone from beginner to experienced in terms of their skill and taste palate. It's called the Green Curve, and it's based on our many years of seeing how our patrons tastes have naturally expanded and evolved.

This book you're holding is also popping with words of wisdom from the people who've come up alongside us on our fifteen-year journey; a colorful cast of inspiring and aspirational characters who use juices and blended drinks every day to fuel their best lives. You'll hear their tips and insights on getting the most from a juicing and blending habit. They range from well-known actors and entertainers to founders of natural beauty companies; from Olympic sprinters and celebrated dancers to filmmakers and chefs. Each one of this diverse group has their own way of using liquid tools: some are devout green juicers who actually crave bitter leaves; others make luscious smoothies enhanced with healthy fats, and many do both, because they've developed an awareness of the kind of nutritional support their body needs at different times. All of them have mastered the art of finding time in their hectic schedules to treat themselves right by making—and yes, sometimes purchasing—vibrantly-colored liquid elixirs, and they unanimously report they feel more centered, clear, creative, and confident as a result.

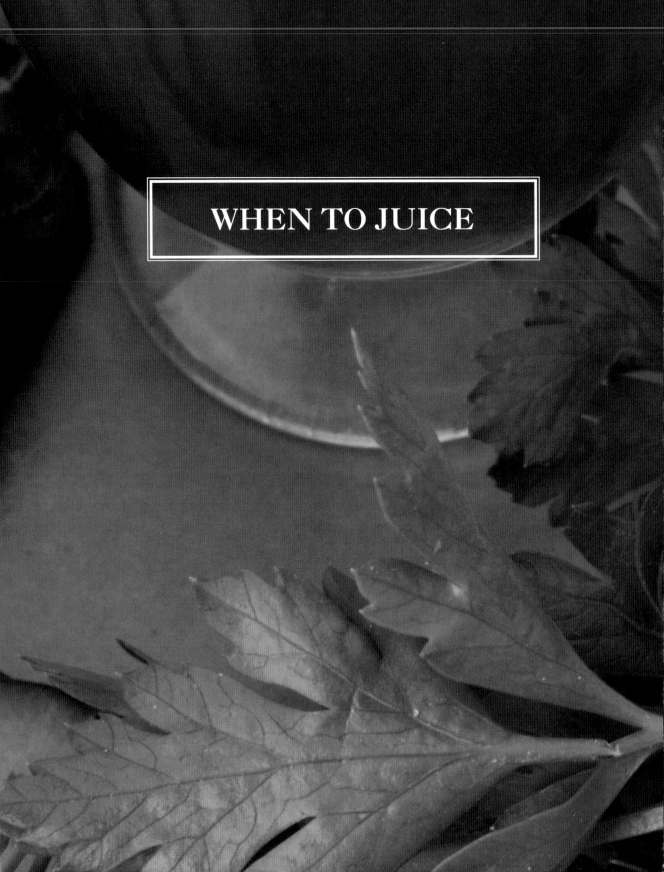

WHEN TO JUICE

EVERY DAY WE HEAR SOME SIMILAR REFRAINS:

"I'm a working mom. I'm always seeking energy and I'm dying to get off the caffeine-crash roller coaster."

"I run out the door in a rush every morning with no time to make a good breakfast, and I fade by midmorning."

"No matter what I eat, I never seem to be satisfied. I'm always grazing, trying to find the thing that will make me feel complete."

"I go from work to a workout, and then commute home, and if I don't replenish properly, I bonk the next day."

"After a long day on the go, the face I see in the mirror looks tired and blah."

DO YOU RECOGNIZE YOURSELF IN ANY OF THESE?

Drinking juices and blends releases the tremendous healing power of raw and living foods, which is why, when you juice and blend regularly, a range of physical ailments—from joint pain, allergies, gut issues, skin problems, mood imbalances, sleep problems, and more—have a chance to improve. This book is designed to help you **lift, clear, glow, nourish,** and **balance.** Here's how.

LIFT

Running your own business is a 24-hour commitment. Juicing is the way I survive on so many levels: It is the easiest breakfast for me to grab and go and it relieves my mind, knowing I filled my body with the right vitamins and minerals to nourish my cells and have taken care of myself first thing in the morning, so I can go forward into my day facing the unexpected. I drink juice first thing because it's the easiest food to digest and run through the system. It feels like I am watering a plant, filling up my body with its live and vibrant life force. And even though I am super dynamic and results oriented, and accomplish a tremendous amount each day, I seem to have a very Zen energy. Maybe it's the juice and food that I put through my body that manifests in my even mood. Ever seen an aggressive yogi? I doubt it. Food really does make a difference.

—Susan Beischel, founder and designer of the luxury natural clothing line Skin; member of the Council of Fashion Designers of America

We are obsessed with the quest for more energy. We're doing more than ever before, constantly out-putting wattage for a never-slow-ing juggle of career and kids, personal dreams, and public ob-ligations. We're pushing harder, working longer—resting less and sleeping worse. Which leaves us in a perpetual net deficit of en-ergy. What are we using to prop ourselves up? Surging quantities of caffeine and chemical-laden, sugar-saturated sodas and en-ergy drinks.

Now, we humbly acknowledge the pleasure of a robust macchi-ato brewed from the finest qual-ity beans, or a delicate oolong steeped to perfection. The prob-lem is when they go from a choice to a dependency. We're relying on these buzzy beverages as liquid life support, but the foundation of energy they provide is rickety. Their initial rush gives way to a crash that undermines us like a trapdoor, and eventually they can take a system-wide toll, acidifying

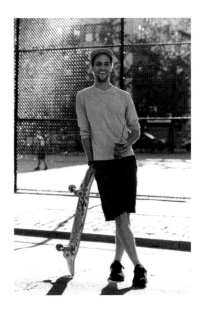

our systems and burning out adre-nal glands. Used in this excessive way, caffeine can be dirty energy: destructive and unsustainable.

Juicing provides a different kind of lift: Think of it as clean power—a more sustainable resource. A glass of juice floods your body with a mother lode of components that are essential to life, giving you a boost of vitality in about 20 minutes. The nutrients are rap-idly absorbed because juicing and blending breaks down the whole plant food and partially "predigests" it. This saves your body some of the energy needed for breaking down solid foods, meaning you intake more nutri-ents with less energy expenditure. Better yet, because the foods are still in their raw, uncooked state, their enzymes are intact and able to lend their full power to your cells, assisting your body in per-forming all the actions it takes to keep you alive. Cells are our tiny energy-producing factories that need oxygen and nutrients and

support for detoxification. In re-turn, they make ATP, the energy that supports life. Give them more of what they need—elements rich in oxygen like chlorophyll from green plants and important mi-cronutrients, and it's not surprising that you feel an extra tingle inside. This is one of the reasons that raw food is so important: It literally fires you up.

JUICING JARGON

Raw food means food that has not been heated above 115°F, which keeps all the bioavailable nutrients intact and in their original state, so you get the richest infusion of nature's bounty.

Living food is a loosely used term that often refers to seeds that are sprouting or just bursting into growth and thus considered ultra full of natural life force. Some people use the term to refer to just-picked vegetables and fruits.

Blending has some other energy benefits. Where juice delivers an instant uplifting boost, partly because there's no tough material for the digestive system to break down, a blended drink has a slower-absorbing quality and the potential to deliver longer-lasting fuel because it contains plenty of fiber, and often, fats and proteins. It is a meal in a cup that has the potential, if you build it right, to carry you all the way from breakfast through to lunch.

We're not going to lie: A raw juice or smoothie won't get you wired like a double latte does. Consider it a different kind of lift, one that nourishes and sustains, perking you up more gently without the jagged takeoff and bumpy landing of caffeine. Some people say that drinking juice feels like "lighting up" their circuitry, and many say their morning habit helps to tone down a reliance on coffee or tea without a great struggle. A green juice or smoothie first thing can help soften the habit of even a hardened espresso denizen.

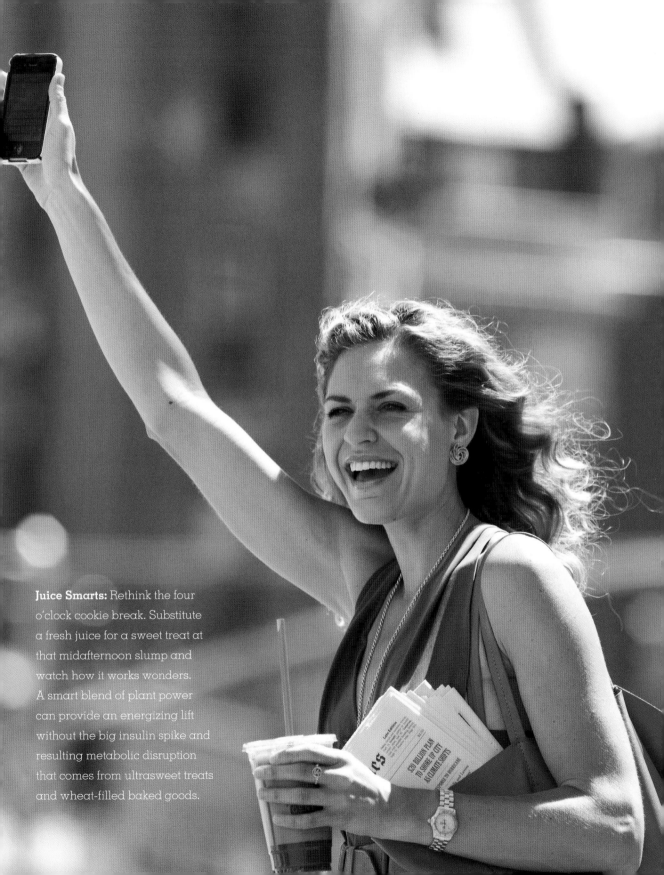

Juice Smarts: Rethink the four o'clock cookie break. Substitute a fresh juice for a sweet treat at that midafternoon slump and watch how it works wonders. A smart blend of plant power can provide an energizing lift without the big insulin spike and resulting metabolic disruption that comes from ultrasweet treats and wheat-filled baked goods.

CLEAR

The residue of modern living and eating can show itself in the guise of a foggy mind, a weighed down body, and a dumpy spirit. Luckily, juicing and blending can bring some levity to the situation. Consider it a 21st-century survival tool that can help you stay buoyed, alert, and feeling bright and clear, even in the gunkiest moments.

This clarity is due in large part to the ways that vegetables (particularly green ones) and some fruits (like grapefruits) deliver potent nutrients that support your on-board cleaning crew, your detoxification system—especially the liver, where most of your detoxification occurs. In addition, the load on your digestive system decreases when you periodically have a liquid snack or meal instead of denser food. This diverts energy away from digestion and toward detoxification, the never-ending cleansing the body does to rid itself of the unavoidable by-products of living (called metabolic wastes) and unwanted toxins from outside. Combined with the greater amounts of fiber moving through your intestines and the highly efficient hydration that comes from juices and blendeds, which help your intestines to eliminate more regularly, you get to enjoy the lighter and brighter effects of improved daily cleansing.

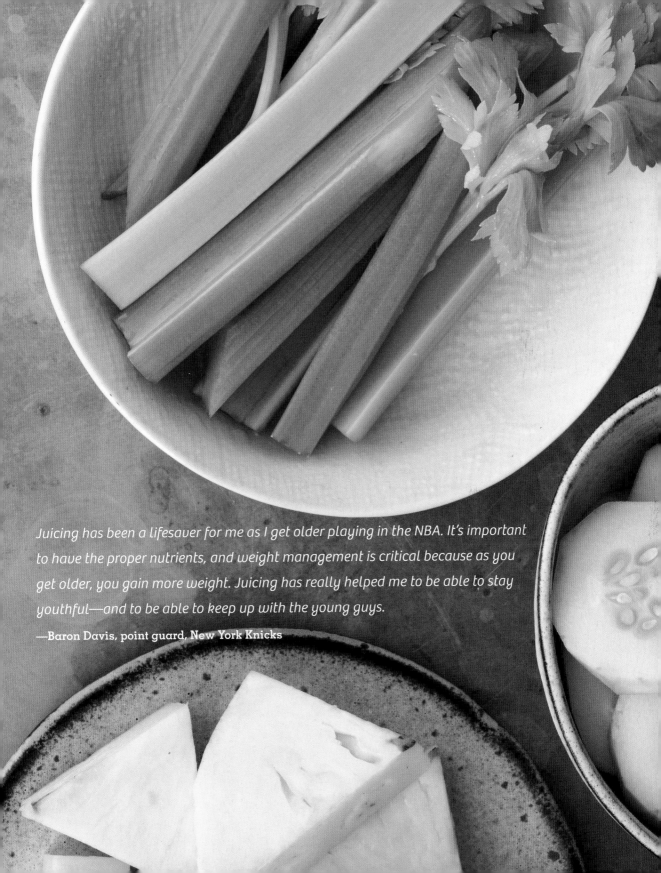

Juicing has been a lifesaver for me as I get older playing in the NBA. It's important to have the proper nutrients, and weight management is critical because as you get older, you gain more weight. Juicing has really helped me to be able to stay youthful—and to be able to keep up with the young guys.

—Baron Davis, point guard, New York Knicks

JUICY TIP

When you feel weighed down or extra sluggish, try doing one day of a liquid morning and evening—a healthy smoothie in the morning and a juice in the evening, or vice versa. This quick "reset" lightens the load on your digestion and helps you sleep better, too.

Equally as important, when these liquid treats integrate themselves into your diet they tend to take the place of convenience foods and snacks like gluten-filled breads, breakfast cereal, baked goods, and pasteurized dairy—all things that have notoriously clogging, dulling, and irritating effects. This gradual reduction in toxifying foods helps you achieve an increasingly detoxified state, because you're eliminating the triggers that cause inflammatory and immune responses. That's why with juices in your life you feel energized, more clear and focused, and, often, more optimistic.

Will all this detoxification affect your waistline? Maybe so, because you're replacing toxic foods that puff you up, due to their inflammatory effect, with a lot more healing whole foods that help you run a cleaner engine. That said, health and well-being is the goal, and weight changes are an added bonus.

Juice Smarts: Studies show that when used in conjunction with a low-glycemic diet, green and veggie juices help to enhance weight loss. Low-glycemic indicates foods with carbohydrates that break down slowly, releasing their glucose (sugar) more gradually into the bloodstream, helping create better blood sugar control and blood-lipid levels, and making you feel more full.

WHAT IS PRESSED OR COLD-PRESSED JUICE?

Cold-pressed juices are the turbo-charged model of juicing, developed specifically for use in cleansing and healing programs. They're made using a labor-intensive process involving a hydraulic press that slowly extracts even higher levels of nutrients from the produce than regular domestic blenders, with extremely low exposure to air. Their major benefit is that they create a completely pulp-free elixir, which floods the body with nutrients without any energy expenditure used on digestion, and can retain full nutritional value for at least three days. That's why they first came to fame through use in intensive healing programs for acute health issues, when the body's capacity is unusually compromised and has almost no extra power to digest and absorb.

In the last few years, cold-pressed juices earned cachet for their use in preventive healthcare programs—multiday detoxification and cleansing programs—because they give the digestive system such a profound break and because many say these juices have the most intense flavors due to their extraordinary extraction capacity. Now cold-press juice has become an everyday drink, and many juice boutiques exclusively sell these ultrafine pressed juices, which they make off site every morning and sell in bottles at premium prices (due to the unavoidably slower production). At Juice Generation we offer both made-to-order centrifugal juices and cold-pressed bottled versions because it's a question of taste and price. Not everyone enjoys pulp-free juice (and sometimes you just want to see your juice made to order before your eyes!).

Can you make cold-pressed juices at home? It requires splurging on a specialized and costly professional-grade machine called a Norwalk Juicer. For most people, a good-quality consumer-level juicer, which extracts juice through crushing and grinding fruits and vegetables, suffices. It delivers plenty of raw nutrients at an efficient speed and cost.

JUICING JARGON

Enzymes are catalysts that regulate every chemical reaction in our cells, enabling all the activities in our body, including digestion and healing. They're abundant in raw foods and their unique shape is damaged by heat and cooking, which is why it's important, especially as we age, to get lots of raw foods in your diet, to help up the supply of enzymes.

Vitamins are organic compounds that the body must get from food and the sun. We require 13 of them: Nine are water soluble (eight B vitamins and C) and four are fat soluble (A, C, E, and K). Cooking foods tends to reduce their vitamin content. Some plants, like broccoli, release more vitamins when steamed.

Minerals are absorbed from the soil by plants and turned into compounds that our tissues can absorb. Plants thus provide us with essential macro minerals like calcium and potassium, as well as trace minerals needed in tiny amounts, like chromium, copper, iron, and zinc.

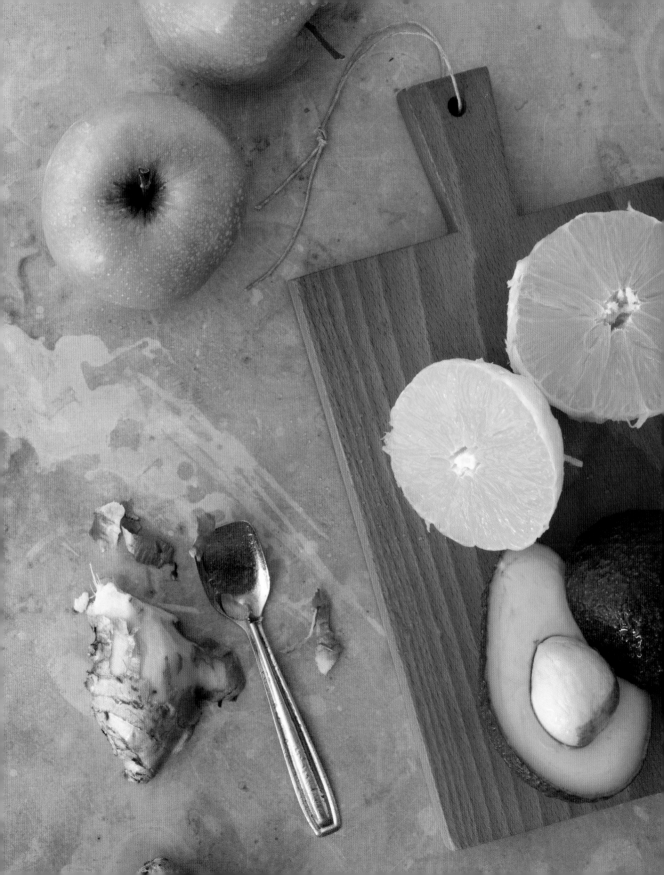

Antioxidants are molecules that help keep us healthy by neutralizing free radicals—highly reactive molecules that damage and degenerate our tissues and cause our bodies to age. Free radicals are produced by our bodies as waste and also enter us via external pollution and toxicity, and even sunlight! Plants have multiple complexes of different neutralizing antioxidants, including Vitamins A, C, and E, and a host of enzymes.

Phytochemicals are the thousands of miraculous and mysterious substances in plants that give them their color, flavor, and aroma. Some, like beta-carotene, resveratrol, curcumin, and lycopene, have been shown to have potent benefits for health and beauty. Many of them are powerful antioxidants.

Electrolytes are substances that become ions in solution and have the ability to conduct electricity. They need to be in optimal balance for our bodies to work well. Sodium and potassium are two that tend to be out of balance in the Standard American Diet—too much sodium, too little potassium. This causes us to wilt like a plant, and can push blood pressure up. Juicing helps to flood our cells with higher potassium, from vegetables like cucumbers and celery, which helps us excrete sodium and return us to our energized best.

Micronutrients refer to all the organic compounds such as vitamins, minerals, and phytochemicals that our bodies need in tiny amounts in order to run properly. Deprived of enough of these micronutrients, we become susceptible to diseases and DNA damage. Folic acid, iron, zinc, iodine, and magnesium are just a few of these wonder substances that nature provides through food.

Fiber is a carbohydrate that is not digested by the body. It can be soluble or insoluble—both are essential for optimal health. Insoluble fiber—found in dark leafy greens, fruit skin, and seeds and nuts—regulates bowl movements and helps to maintain a healthy pH balance in the intestines, which can prevent colon cancer. Soluble fiber—found in fruit pulps, bananas, some nuts, flaxseeds, beans, avocados, blueberries, cucumbers, and more—helps you feel full longer, which regulates blood sugar levels. Soluble fiber can also lower LDL cholesterol by disrupting the absorption of dietary cholesterol.

Omega-3 and omega-6 fatty acids are essential fatty acids that we do not produce—they can only be obtained from our diet. Omega-3s are made up of two fatty acids, EPA and DHA, which are the basis of the hormones that control immune function, blood clotting, and cell growth. There are limited sources—cold water fish (like salmon), avocados, walnuts, and flaxseeds (vegetarian sources contain ALA, a precursor omega-3 that the body must convert to EPA and DHA). Most people tend to have low levels of this essential fatty acid, which is where blended drinks full of these good plant foods can help.

The best vegetables for skin are made up of mostly water, which instantly hydrates the skin for a gorgeous glow. One of my absolute favorite drinks is the classic, all-green juice of kale, spinach, parsley, cucumber, celery, lemon, and ginger. All of these ingredients benefit the skin with the ultimate hydration and more. Kale has vitamin K, which helps brighten your complexion and reduce dark circles. Kale and spinach also have vitamin A, which encourages your skin to repair itself and retain moisture. Parsley is a natural deodorizer that has many vital vitamins that keep your immune system strong, and you'll rejuvenate and refresh the body and nourish the skin with celery. Cucumbers contain vitamin C and are rich in caffeic acid, which helps soothe the skin. They also contain silica, which contributes to collagen formation. (Try to buy organic cucumber, since silica is mostly on the skin and this can be added to the juice.) Lemon helps in the detoxification process of the body, but it can also be used directly on the skin as a natural exfoliator. Ginger acts as an anti-inflammatory in the body to keep you going during a busy time.

To replenish the skin, coconut water contains vitamins, minerals, and electrolytes that taste delicious! And aloe water is an amazing detoxifier that provides collagen and elastin repair for healthy skin.

—Pat McGrath, makeup artist and beauty guru

GLOW

Nutraceutical beauty is today's booming trend; it features luxurious face products with active nutrients and supplements from food sources that nourish the skin, give it a radiant look, and help slow aging. Juice is the original nutraceutical, and works from the inside out, helping to diminish wrinkles and develop dewier and clearer skin, brighter, whiter eyes, and a distinctive "juice glow." The rejuvenating effect of consuming vegetables, especially greens, is partly due to their alkalizing effect, which helps to balance out the acidity in our tissues that is a common effect of our modern life and diet and that can lead to skin disorders like acne, rosacea, and a generally dull, dry complexion. Then there are the high levels of naturally occurring antioxidants you consume, which help combat the aging effects of pollution and environmental stress and help create healthy and more vibrant skin.

Add in the fact that the electrolytes in juices deliver hydration that has an undeniably energizing effect on the skin, and we are confident to issue a challenge: Get back to us after a week of juicing and blending your cucumbers, celery, and spinach, and tell us your face doesn't look better. Don't forget to check your hair and nails, too: When they receive good doses of minerals like zinc, copper, thiamin, niacin, and iron, along with good proteins like the sulfur-bearing amino acids methionine, cysteine, and cystine (which are found in spirulina and super seeds like hemp), your locks and talons will get extra strong and shiny.

NOURISH

Blended foods pack a lot of nutrient density into a very small package. People think that they need a lot of food to feel good, but it's not about volume, it's about density. In a 16- or 32-ounce blended drink, you are getting so much dense nutrition in a small volume.

—Jason Wrobel, chef and host of the Cooking Channel's
  How to Live to 100

Everyone knows they're supposed to pack their diets full of plant-based food to stay healthy; the question is, "How on earth do I do that every single day?" Nine daily servings of fruits and vegetables are considered a minimum baseline for health (which means 2 cups fruit and 2½ cups vegetables, but up that number considerably if you require a caloric intake higher than 2000 calories a day). Blitzing salad bowl–size servings of leaves, stalks, fruits, and roots into liquid form is one way to achieve that goal; reducing them into such a concentrated form delivers a large nutritional punch in a small amount of food.

Think of it as flipping on its head that all-American logic, that size matters and we need to eat massive portions in order to function. So much of the modern diet is super sized but nutritionally empty.

A smartly constructed smoothie packs an abundance of good things into one glass. Think: giant handfuls of fresh vegetables and fruits; nutrient-dense superseeds like hemp and chia, and nuts for good fats and protein; and even functional ingredients (natural ingredients that have specific physical and mental enhancing effects, like turmeric root or cinnamon). These all give you extra help where you need it, like lifting the mood or calming inflammation. It's an exercise in elegant simplicity. Some of nature's greatest foods give their effects in small and potent amounts.

Which is why juicing and blending can help to counter the modern dilemma: We're eating more food than ever before, but our bodies are still deprived of essential nutrients due to the industrialized way that our foods are grown, produced, and processed. If you use the freshest, organic-whenever-possible, and local-whenever-possible produce, which research shows has higher amounts of essential micronutrients, you can replenish some key factors that your diet may be missing, clearing out obstacles to feeling, looking, and performing at your best.

Don't forgo food: Wise juicing and blending means using liquid foods as supplements and enhancements to your diet, not ditching your regular meals. But in the quest to be vital and vibrant, it's not always volume of food we're after; it's nutritional density.

Juice Smarts: One cup of carrot or celery juice provides most of the same nutrients found in about 4 to 5 cups of the same vegetables in whole form. (Different juicers produce different amounts.)

THE SUGAR QUESTION

Smart juicing means becoming savvy about sugars in your drinks. Successful long-term juicers learn to liquefy greens and vegetables on a daily basis, and to juice sweet-tasting fruits and the sweetest root vegetables, which are higher in natural sugars, in moderation.

"But these are naturally occurring sugars in my pineapple, mango, and beets!" you say. "How can they be bad?" The truth is that ultrasweet fruits and sweet root vegetables are dense sources of polysaccharide carbohydrates, which when digested or broken down in juice turn into glucose and other simple sugars. This isn't too problematic when you eat the whole plant with its fiber intact, because it's a slow process to break down the entire mass and extract the sugar out. But when you juice them and take out the fibers, the sugars are delivered to the bloodstream in a much faster manner, causing a bigger sugar rush and a larger insulin spike (insulin is the hormone that regulates sugars in the blood). The sugars, if not used up right away in vigorous activity, get stored as fat; the insulin spike, if it happens repeatedly, disrupts your metabolism, with weight problems or blood sugar–related illnesses a possible result.

That's why ensuring your liquid meals frequently feature greens and low-sugar fruits like berries or tart green apples is a key to a healthy juicing and blending habit. Getting your greens is at the very heart of the Juice Generation's ethos: They are alkalinizing, anti-inflammatory, chlorophyll-packed gifts from Mother Nature. Adding healthy fats to your drinks, in the form of avocados, seeds, nut butters, or even via flax oil or coconut stirred into fresh-made juice, can also be a tool to slow down the speed of sugars entering your bloodstream and achieve good balance.

If you are overweight or have high blood pressure, diabetes, or high cholesterol, be even more vigilant about limiting your sweet fruits and pure root-vegetable drinks until you normalize these conditions.

JUICE IMPOSTERS

Supermarket shelves and convenience store coolers are stocked with bottled, packaged, and frozen juices and smoothies. So why bother to make your drinks fresh at home? Because most of these items are juice imposters! Most of the "juice" beverages filling store shelves are several steps away from the raw, whole foods they came from—and the ingredients they contain are not always benign.

Almost all store-bought juices are pasteurized at high heat to kill off any potential pathogens in the juice and give it a long shelf life (up to a year if unopened!). This sterilizing process also, not surprisingly, kills off the fragile enzymes and a lot of the active power of the vitamins and antioxidants. Your fruit or vegetable nectar goes from fresh to, well, somewhat vapid. Pasteurization does enable big food producers to make huge amounts of product and ship it nationwide without fear that contaminants are left in, but the ones who benefit the most from this process are the producers, not the consumers, who are left to guzzle drinks stripped of their best components. We'd rather wash our produce well, juice it fresh and turbo-charged to get all the nutritional and energetic benefits—and watch it degrade naturally like nature intended if we forget to drink it.

═ READY MADE JUICES: ═ OUR ADVISORY SYSTEM

CODE YELLOW: Bottled smoothies and juices with "no added sugars." These convenience-store quick fixes look healthy, with their cute labels covered in fruits (and maybe vegetables), but they're less than fresh. The popular ones may say "all natural," but they're rarely organic. Plus, check the ingredient list and the nutritional content. Each 15-ounce bottle might contain two servings; and if it's a fruit-only juice, the whole bottle may have 50 grams of sugars from carbohydrates. (Compare to an ultra-green juice you make at home that may contain just 2 grams.) Bottled "green" smoothies are often mainly fruit with a touch of green. If you're going to have one, read the fine print, water down if possible, and consume the contents in small increments.

CODE ORANGE: Bottled or frozen juices partly or fully "made from concentrate." This process heats the juice to evaporate water and separate out the pulp, concentrating the flavorings, and then recombines the concentrate and pulp to achieve the concentration and flavor the producer desires. This concentrate is then stored in refrigerated tanks until it can be packaged or reconstituted. Along the way, the heating process pasteurizes the juice. Though many argue there's nothing inherently bad about a concentrate if it has no added sugars or flavorings—again, you're drinking a lot of the quick-hit carbs without the advantages of fresh juice's life force.

CODE RED: "Juice cocktails" or "juice drinks." Three words: *Back away slowly.* And, when it comes to your kids: *Just say no.* These beverages may have fruit-derived ingredients, but they're so concentrated and enhanced they are essentially sugar water delivering empty, and damaging, calories. With up to 20 teaspoons of sugar per bottle, they're as bad as the sugariest sodas! (We noticed that a certain grape beverage from one of America's favorite brands has 72 grams of sugar, the same as six scoops of ice-cream; and a canned tea beverage we cannot name, with two fruits in its name, contains 84 grams of sugar!)

STATUS PENDING

Some supermarkets are starting to carry bottles of cold-pressed juice; but they're a different animal from the cold-pressed juices sold in juiceries, which have a three-day life if unopened. The supermarket juices have been pasteurized to survive transit and have a much longer shelf life. This is done through a new process called High Pressure Processing (or High Pressure Pascalization) that, its advocates say, keeps most of the fragile nutrients intact, because the process does not use heat. Rather, it surrounds the packaged juice in water at high pressure.

Yet when you pick up one of these juices, you simply don't know how long it's been on the shelf. Four days? Ten days? Fourteen? HPP is helping large companies ramp up their distribution, but we're not fans. We think it's processed juice masquerading as fresh. Crack one of these beverages open and see: The taste and vibrancy will be different from the juice made right before your eyes. That said, in a pinch, if you're yearning for a juice and there's no made-to-order juicery within reach, these bottles are by far your best bet.

YOUR BEST STRATEGY

Make your own juices and smoothies and watch them come directly from nature's own container: the whole fruit or vegetable in its untouched state.

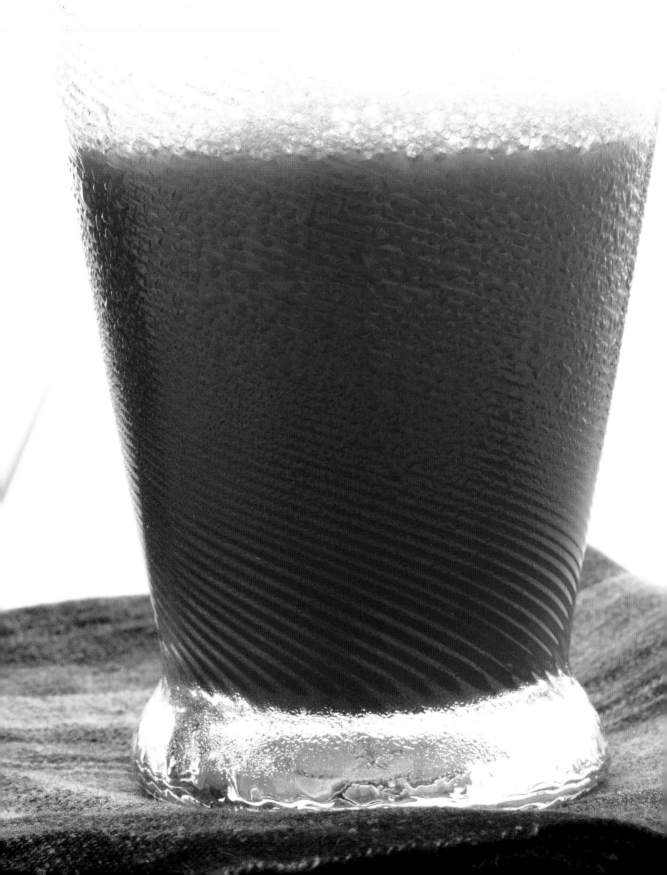

= BALANCE =

Dynamic members of the Juice Generation know that life doesn't have a lot of wiggle room. Staying healthy, with fewer illnesses and colds, is critical when you're juggling many balls in the air. Who's going to catch you if you fall? Juicing mavens use juicing and blending as their secret weapon for staying in balance. It boosts the immune system, making it a preventive healthcare boon. It protects against pain and chronic disease by alkalizing your blood, which buffers the acidic imbalance from sugars, meat, dairy, and grains that is a major cause of joint and muscle pain and a gateway into degenerative disease.

Juicing and blending also helps create a more balanced relationship to food. Ardent juicers report a reduction in cravings and say their appetite feels under control. At a fundamental level, the body is more nourished, and when it's replete with the nutrients it needs, it sends signals to the brain that it is well fed. Satiety—the happy feeling of having had enough to eat and drink—is increased by consuming vibrant flavors along with healthy fats. Have some almonds with your juice, or put some coconut oil in your smoothie, and it's easier than you can imagine to get that satisfaction.

Even fearsome sugar cravings have a chance to simmer down, or even dissolve, when sugary addictions are replaced with fresh juices or green drinks. Cravings usually come from an overgrowth of candida living in the guts, which feeds on sugar and tells you to consume more. If you ditch 4 o'clock cookies and spontaneous candy attacks in favor of healthier fare, these hungry demons can begin to die off, and bother you less.

Many renowned healing centers and methods use juicing as a tool for more serious conditions: There are green juicing programs designed to reverse type 2 diabetes and cancer patients have found success in a somewhat controversial healing system called Gerson Therapy, which follows a strict regime of using 14 cold-pressed juices a day to help their bodies heal.

JUICE VS. BLEND

Though some people take sides—juicy fruit and veggie elixirs versus thick, luscious purees—we prefer an equal opportunity approach. We like to juice, blend, and eat our vegetables and fruits—raw and cooked. This is about having *more* options, not less.

The number one perk of choosing juice over blends: Nutrients are easily absorbed because the foods are virtually predigested; the resulting energetic uplift can have a supercharge effect. The cons are that you've taken the fiber out, which can have your hungry tummy seeking solid food soon after the last sip; and, if you overdo the fruits, you'll get a quick sugar spike, which as a daily habit isn't ideal because it contributes to weight gain and insulin destabilization. If you end up predominantly juicing, be sure your diet is filled with *lots* of good fiber—don't use the juices as an excuse not to eat vegetables or fiber-rich whole foods. And don't go bananas putting only sweet stuff in your juicer!

The pros of blending are that you leave all the fiber in the drink, which most people don't have enough of in their diets, and you can easily blend in healthy fats and sources of protein to make your drink more of a meal. The cons for some people is the texture—thicker, obviously, which some love but others don't enjoy—and the not-quite-the-same instant infusion to the cells as juice, because of the fiber. (This is why juices, which don't require any work by your digestive system to break down the components, are used in healing and restorative juice-cleansing programs.)

— PEACE, LOVE AND JUICE! —

Slow down. Take a breath. Chop carrots. Juicing is a kind of mindfulness training. The act of handling your food deliberately—washing it, cutting it, and watching it transform with a rush of flavor and aroma and a flood of color—has the power to stop your mind from racing and connect you to the present. Bring your awareness to the tangy, succulent tastes in your mouth as you drink, and you cannot help but grin. It's a moment of respite.

OK, so the whole experience might just last a few minutes—and then it's back to the rat race. But consider it a food meditation of sorts. Anecdotal evidence suggests that the juice habit has a happifying effect—it floods contentment, as well as nutrition, through your veins.

It's also empowering. Making a juice or healthy smoothie is one of the easiest ways to pave your way to your and your family's good health and to getting more intimate with the energy of what you eat. Food's gotten far too hands-off in recent decades: The shift to eating prepared meals, grocery-store dinners, and restaurant food makes everyone feel a little grief. What happened, we find ourselves wondering on our commute or work break, to having the time to cook with joy and love?

We say: It starts with the simple and short act of pulverizing a rainbow of colors, sprinkling in a hint of spice or a splash of citrus, and serving it joyously to yourself or someone you care about. A world of discovery opens up through juicing to deliver that happifying

effect: You savor a plethora of natural flavors you have never known before; learn the pleasure of buying produce that's in season from local markets and get to know who grows it; and, by gaining an awareness of what nature's up to month by month, have a new appreciation for your place in the greater whole.

For many people, juicing and blending is a doorway into a bigger lifestyle shift that includes eating consciously, shopping responsibly, and living in a more wakeful way to the natural world. It's a way of getting back to basics and being more attuned to body and soul.

Welcome to the Juice Generation!

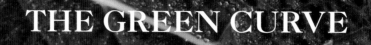

THE GREEN CURVE

I'm a juicing addict! I've been searching for ways to optimize every facet of my mind, body, and physical performance. The benefits of juicing have opened up doors to a sharper mind, a more powerful and explosive body, and an overall feeling of wellness. I'm hooked—and I'm never going back!

—Steve Weatherford, Super Bowl champion
   and New York Giants punter

The Green Curve is a step-by-step journey into a new food world that is simple, fun, and satisfying while helping you integrate raw juices and sumptuous smoothies into your life at a natural pace.

It's based on years of real-life observations at our stores: First-time customers tend to start with drinks on the sweeter, fruitier side, eyeing the greener drinks from a distance. A few visits later, they get more curious, venture outside their comfort zones, and experiment with one of the sweeter green juices, like a watermelon-kale. (Typical response: "You can't even taste the kale!")

Convinced by the refreshing uplift they've found, they eventually go the whole nine yards and pick up an ultra-green concoction—one of our detoxifying drinks filled with seven kinds of leafy, liquidy greens, with only a splash of lemon added. They might get adventurous and add a shot of wheatgrass—a health elixir bursting with living energy—or green-blue algae full of vitamins, minerals, amino acids, and fatty acids.

Some weeks or months after first coming in, our new recruits discover a new range to their palate that didn't exist before, and they've successfully developed a "happy green habit"—an ingrained desire to give their body what will serve it best. (And it explains why these days, our green drinks outsell fruit-only offerings by ten to one.)

When it comes to getting started in your own kitchen, this unfolding can happen in the same way. There are a couple of other factors to consider as well. Learning to carve out extra time in your day, starting with simple and nonintimidating recipes, and keeping costs within your budget are equally important. The Green Curve addresses all these by guiding you at a comfortable gait from simple juicing and blending recipes to more sophisticated ones. You'll start with basic juice or blended combos with sweeter profiles that you can make easily and quickly from minimal ingredients. You'll progress to recipes with more ingredients and a medium-green profile—half savory, half sweet. Then, if you choose, you'll explore exotic options that throw in exciting new ingredients that tend to have the greenest flavors yet and that might require a few more purchases and prep steps.

Juice Smarts: The more intensely colored a fruit or vegetable is, the more chemically active antioxidants it usually contains. Go bright!

Don't worry. This isn't a severe self-help program—*30 Days to a Much Improved You, If You Give Up Everything You Love*. It's about discovery. A happy green habit that lasts is founded on a genuine love for the flavors, textures, colors, and possibilities of vibrant, plant-based ingredients, and is based on enjoying the process of combining them in exciting new ways. The Green Curve helps you to develop this love by presenting sumptuous treats alongside the good-for-you drinks, and keeping you jazzed with a spectrum of flavors, from sweet to rich to tart to tangy. You'll use old standards in new ways—the cucumber is a lot cooler than you ever realized—and discover some of the new juicing and blending-world trends to impress your friends. (Clue: It's where fresh coconuts meet superfruits.)

WHAT IS GREEN?

The Green Curve is designed to ease you into consuming more of the leafy and dark green plants that pack such extraordinary health power. To us, green is an umbrella word describing all things vibrantly phytonutrient-filled—full of plant power. We use the term a little loosely: It involves all the foods that are actually green—from spinach and celery to kale, watercress, lettuce, and more—as well as ones that are all the other colors of the rainbow: from orange, yellow, and red to purple, blue, and brown. Green means natural; green means plant-based; green means full of earth's powerful energizing and healing power.

MAKING YOUR WAY UP THE CURVE

The Green Curve rolls out our favorite recipes over three distinct phases that we recommend should last for about three weeks each. This 3 x 3 formula helps you get accustomed to the recipes in each phase at a reasonable pace before moving on to the next level of complexity and flavor intensity.

PHASE 1: You'll aim to make two to three juices or smoothies a week, with at least 30 percent including a handful of leafy greens like spinach or kale.

PHASE 2: You'll aim to make five juices or smoothies a week, at least 50 percent including handfuls of leafy greens.

PHASE 3: You'll aim to have a drink with green vegetables in it every day, with a few non-green elixirs as needed or as treats! That's a 90 percent green rate.

The goal throughout the Green Curve is also to start listening to your body and noticing how different types of things affect you and what you might naturally feel drawn to consume at different moments.

There are no hard and fast rules. If you're ready to dial it up after one week on Phase 1 and dive into the new ingredients of Phase 2, or would rather start at Phase 2 because you're already adept, go ahead; and if you want to linger longer than three weeks, feel free.

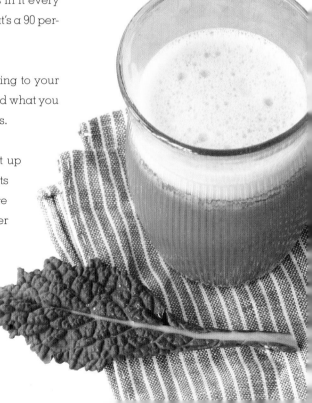

ADJUSTING TO GREENS

WARNING: YOUR PALATE HAS BEEN HIJACKED!

Why can the initial sips of good-for-you drinks be challenging? We'll admit what most juice books don't tell you: Though the greener, more veggie-heavy drinks on the spectrum become second nature when you get in the groove, that initial hit may shock your taste buds. The reality is that green-y, leafy, cruciferous-y, healing-herb–filled drinks are not exactly the mainstay of the Standard American Diet that most of us were raised on, and their flavor profiles are almost the complete opposite of what we recognize as "yummy!" The mind knows they're good for us; the mouth rejects this wisdom.

If this is your experience, it is OK. It is because your palate has been hijacked!

Consider that even the healthiest person is biologically conditioned to crave non-green flavors. Did you know every one of your tongue's 10,000 taste buds is wired to detect sugar, and each hit of the sweet stuff activates our brain's pleasure centers? In fact, the human tongue can detect four flavors—salt, sour, bitter, and sweet—but we're more naturally drawn to sweet because we've evolved from primate ancestors whose entire survival M.O. was to plunder super-ripe sweet fruits in trees—the best source of energy and water for a busy primate.

And since those early days—through no fault of your own—that tendency has become more pronounced, as humans developed agriculture, grains, and the ability to produce dense, carbohydrate-filled food. The natural sweet tooth has gotten more exaggerated. (By the way, if you think the primate diet sounds about right, consider that our chimp friends are always in active mode, swinging on branches, burning through carbohydrates at rapid speed, not perched all day in front of a computer screen, storing up carbs as fat.)

Our pleasure centers are also fired up by fatty, salty things, because we need fat as well as the right amounts of sodium to survive. Now factor in how our taste buds have been taken on a wild ride over the last few decades. Big corporations have figured out how to exploit our natural palate by developing edible products that deliver artificially enhanced instant gratification to our neuro pleasure centers.

The good news is that taste bud preferences can change and palates can transform. When you consume less of the dominant flavor profiles found in sweet and processed foods and gradually add in new flavors found in fresh, green, tart, and leafy ones, a kind of "waking up" occurs. Your palate literally expands. As the loud noise of artificially enhanced foods dies down, you gain a heightened awareness of the subtler yet delightful flavors naturally found in fruits, vegetables, nuts, seeds, and sprouts.

PRODUCE MYTH BUSTED

MYTH: Fresh vegetables cost more than protein-dense foods.

Fresh veggies and fruits can seem pricier than their meaty counterparts, but USDA studies have found that, pound-for-pound, produce is actually less expensive than most protein-rich foods and processed foods. One of the keys to mastering affordable juicing and blending is to seek out alternative places to buy in volume, and to be flexible according to seasonable availability. When your favorite summer vegetables are out-of-season and getting shipped in from afar, consider switching to a smoothie with frozen fruits.

———

GOT TIME TO CHECK EMAIL? YOU'VE GOT TIME TO JUICE.

Buying your ingredients; washing and storing them; chopping and juicing or blending them; and inevitably, cleaning the juicer or blender afterward . . . there's no getting around the fact that juicing and blending involves finding a little extra time. The time factor is why thousands of people bought juicers back in the 80s (along with their roller blades), used them once . . . and then put them in the garage where they're still gathering dust. (And also why the blending trend, with its speedy production and cleanup, is possibly outpacing juicing in its growth.)

Rest assured that things have evolved since those early days: there are juicers on the market that can be cleaned in under 90 seconds; there are after-work farmers' markets and Community Supported Agriculture schemes (CSAs) that make buying your baskets of vegetables and fruits not only affordable, but fun. And with a few expert kitchen tips (like organizing your fridge and washing certain produce in advance), you can streamline the process down to ten minutes—or even five if you're making an ultra simple juice or blended beverage. The Green Curve will get you comfortable carving out a few extra minutes little by little—and not diving in to complex concoctions straight off the bat.

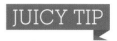

JUICY TIP

When it comes to best price and taste, buying what's in season will reward you most. Get acquainted with the deep flavor of ripe strawberries and tomatoes harvested at their peak, and you might start to question the taste and the sustainability of midwinter versions flown in from afar.

HOW MUCH JUICE IS TOO MUCH JUICE?

The goal of juicing is not to follow a protocol of a specific amount or schedule. The goal is to find what suits you and makes you feel good. Pay attention to your body and don't follow a set of rules that works for someone else. When in doubt, remember less is more. Start with a glass of juice or a small smoothie, and try it out first thing in the morning if you can. Make sure that you keep eating a healthy solid-food diet, even if you occasionally substitute a liquid meal for a plated meal. If you find you want to increase the number of liquid meals in your day, be sure to include lots of green, vegetable-rich drinks, coconut waters, and nut milks, and keep fruits in check.

Though the Green Curve is not a cleanse, some enhanced detoxification may occur, especially if you are also shifting off of irritating or toxifying foods. This could express itself as greater energy and better bowel movements, but also as temporary headaches and fatigue. Many healers say that the three-month mark is when people begin to notice deep and lasting changes from true dietary improvement. Three months happens to be the lifespan of red blood cells, so perhaps putting vibrant foods into your body for that length of time, along with cutting out bad habits, is why 90 days is a marker for a substantial shift. So consider making your Green Curve journey three months of adventure and exploration!

JUICE DIY: GETTING YOUR KITCHEN PREPPED

Do you need a kitchen remodel to join the juice generation? Not at all. A couple of pieces of equipment—which you may already own—and some savvy shopping skills will get you started. If purchasing a juicer is too much of a leap at first, in Phase 1 you can begin with a blender and acquire a juicer later.

———

SPOTLIGHT: THE JUICER

There are two kinds of juicers for at-home juicing. **Centrifugal juicers** grind produce to a pulp and release the juice by spinning it through a serrated metal basket at an extremely high speed. **Masticating juicers** "chew" the produce slowly, by pushing it through a slow-moving drill and squeezing out the juice. Centrifugals tend to be cheaper and are considerably faster at their job. Masticating juicers have their own advantage: Their slower speed means they don't cause as much friction as centrifugal spinners, meaning less heating up of the produce. Heat will speed up the oxidation of the naturally occurring enzymes and nutrients in the produce that occurs when you chop and break down whole food.

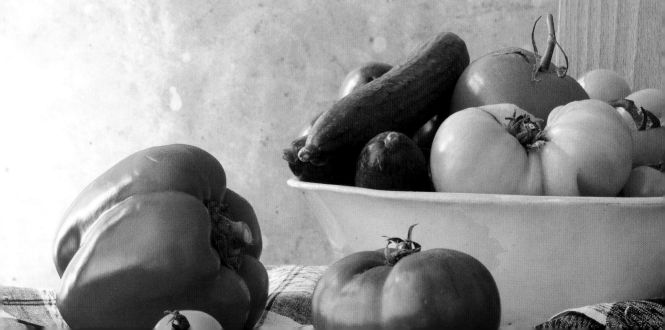

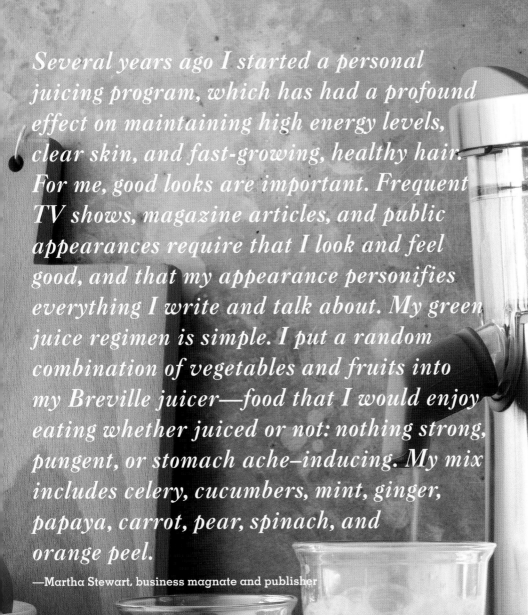

Several years ago I started a personal juicing program, which has had a profound effect on maintaining high energy levels, clear skin, and fast-growing, healthy hair. For me, good looks are important. Frequent TV shows, magazine articles, and public appearances require that I look and feel good, and that my appearance personifies everything I write and talk about. My green juice regimen is simple. I put a random combination of vegetables and fruits into my Breville juicer—food that I would enjoy eating whether juiced or not: nothing strong, pungent, or stomach ache–inducing. My mix includes celery, cucumbers, mint, ginger, papaya, carrot, pear, spinach, and orange peel.

—Martha Stewart, business magnate and publisher

JUICY TIP

Single gear (or "single auger") masticating juicers tend to be more affordable and easier to clean. Twin-gear (or "titrating") models are for devout juicers: They turn even more slowly and are said by juice aficionados to be the most efficient of all and the closest machine to a hydraulic press, though they are costly and will take a little longer to clean. A third at-home option is one of the new dual-extraction juicers that crushes and presses produce at a low speed. Its proponents say it gets even more nutrients than a masticating juicer and does not aerate the produce at all.

Juice Smarts: If you don't already own an electric citrus juicer, you don't need a special one for citrus if you have a juicer. (With a citrus juicer, you also won't get the important nutrients from the white citrus pith the way you will by putting the whole peeled fruit through the juicer.)

A masticator also tends to get more juice out of your vegetables and fruits, especially the essential leafy greens. They can usually extract liquid from delicate plants like wheatgrass and sprouts, where most centrifugals cannot. They are typically more expensive to purchase; however, the benefits reveal themselves over time, when money is saved due to their efficiency with extraction. Other selling points: Many of the "single auger" masticating juicers come apart quickly and are extremely quick to clean. And there are now some vertical masticating juicers that can fit neatly into a snug kitchen corner. The cons: They do juice more slowly, and almost always require that you cut your produce into smaller chunks. If every second counts in your morning, you may want to look for one of the good-quality, speedy centrifugals. When shopping, keep in mind that cheap juicers tend to deliver less volume, and are less durable.

JUICING TIPS

When juicing, keeps these points in mind:

1. Pass your pulp through a second time to extract every ounce of juice from your produce.

2. Centrifugals usually produce more foam in the juice because they are more oxygenated. If foam bothers you, pour juice through a tea strainer and squish it through with a clean finger.

3. Keep a toothbrush by your kitchen sink to clean pulp off your juicer's metal graters.

SHOPPING FOR A JUICER? THESE QUESTIONS ARE KEY

How much do I have to spend right now? Can I afford more upfront and save by getting more out of my produce down the line, or is my budget on the tighter side today?

How long does the juicer take to produce juice—and more critical, to clean? Bothersome cleanup will stop even an enthusiast in their tracks. Check online reviews on every machine to get real-people feedback.

How efficient is the machine at extracting juice? Does it extract a good amount, especially from leaves? Does the pulp come out fairly dry (meaning most of the juice is out) or is it wet and goopy?

How fast or slow does it work, and what are the purported effects on its nutritional quality?

How long is the warranty on the juicer and its parts?

Will it fit on my kitchen counter and how does it look?

SPOTLIGHT: THE BLENDER

Chances are you own a basic blender. That will get you started whipping up blended drinks. But bear in mind that a $20 blender might lack the power to grind frozen fruits, and certainly raw nuts, into pureed or ground form. (A burning smell during operation is a sure sign your blender can't handle it.) Medium-price blenders can do a better job with frozen produce and achieve a good consistency.

The true joy of blending is revealed with high-speed blenders, like those by Vitamix, the grandfather of all blenders, and from its newer rival, Blendtec. These (expensive) workhorses of the professional kitchen have become lusted-over items for amateurs because they are true heavy hitters. The consistency they achieve with blended drinks is remarkable (think: as creamy as a milkshake); they grind nuts and water beautifully into nut milks or instantly turn dry nuts into powder for your smoothie; and they liquidize things very quickly without wear and tear on the machine.

Some small, portable high-speed blenders now exist—often sold on late-night infomercials—that can be especially great for making smoothies at work or on the road. They may not stand up to long-term use in the kitchen like a full-size model, but they achieve surprisingly good consistency.

MORE TOOLS OF THE TRADE

A FEW SIMPLE KITCHEN INSTRUMENTS WILL MAKE DAILY JUICING AND BLENDING A BREEZE.

Cutting boards for chopping produce. Bamboo boards are from sustainable resources, naturally antimicrobial, and cost effective.

Solid chef's knife for chopping. Keep it well sharpened but stored separately from your other kitchenware so as not to dull the blade. Tip: A good chef's knife will work for cracking coconuts safely and efficiently.

Sharp paring knife for opening fruits with hard rinds, like pomegranates.

Metal kitchen bowls for catching nut milk and coconut water.

Plastic spatula, or better yet a coconut scraper or "de-meater," for swiftly getting coconut flesh out.

Nut milk bag, or cheesecloth plus a metal sieve, to make homemade nut milks.

Mason jars or clean, recycled glass food jars.

Biodegradable produce wash and biodegradable detergent. (See page 66 for homemade produce wash recipes.)

Compost pail

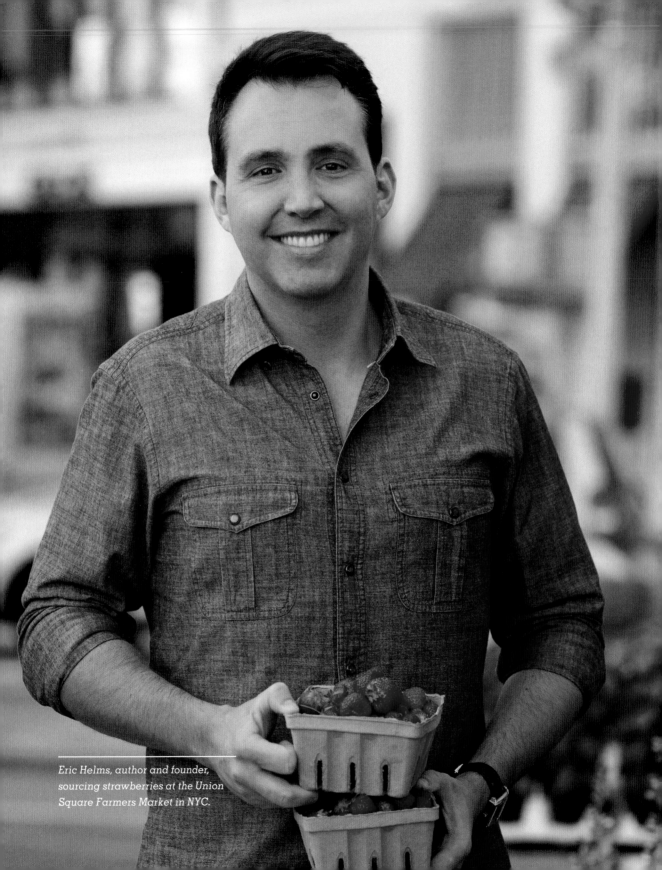

Eric Helms, author and founder,
sourcing strawberries at the Union
Square Farmers Market in NYC.

SHOPPING FOR PRODUCE

When it comes to produce, fresh is best, organic is even better, and local and chemical-free is ideal. We can't wait until the day when every person who wants to can easily and affordably adopt a 100 percent organic kitchen. Until that day comes, here are some ways to make the best choices.

1 If organic produce at your local farmers' market is too costly, look for stalls selling locally grown, pesticide-free produce that may not necessarily be certified organic. Ask the vendors how they farm and what kind of sprays and fertilizers are used. For many small-scale growers, organic certification is prohibitively costly, yet they still refrain from using chemicals either in fertilizing or pest reduction, and their prices are very fair. To find a market in your area, go to localharvest.org.

2 Buy organic for the most pesticide-heavy foods whenever you can. (See Clean Scene, page 63). At Juice Generation, we've always been a stickler for organic greens—these foods suck up so much water, we want them to be clean. Fruits with tougher skins like grapefruit, bananas, pineapples, mangoes, watermelons, and avocados will not contain as many pesticides and other chemicals, so these are less of an urgent concern.

3 Be a bargain shopper. If you find a bumper crop of beautiful organic berries, peaches, cherries, or other soft fruits at a market at their seasonally lowest price, stock up, prep if necessary, and freeze in separate baggies for months of off-season smoothie-making. (You'll find easy directions for freezing fruits successfully online.)

4 Get involved with growing your own. A little digging around may produce surprising resources in your area for helping you to plant an edible garden at home, getting involved in farm volunteer programs, or enrolling your kids in a garden initiative at school. This trend is only going to grow and grow.

5 Wax on, wax off: At the supermarket, check if conventionally grown apples and cucumbers are coated with wax (this seals in their water and keeps them looking fresh during long travel times). These waxes can have pesticides and fungicides added, and don't tend to rinse off with water (which is another reason to have a biodegradable produce wash on hand). You can peel these things, of course—but then you're losing valuable nutrients concentrated in the surface layer. Nix the produce that looks suspiciously shiny.

CLEAN SCENE

The following juicing ingredients tend to be the most chemical-laden when grown conventionally, so grab the organic version whenever possible.

Apples	Bell peppers
Carrots	Celery
Cherries, grapes	Cucumbers
Lettuces	Peaches, nectarines
Pears	Spinach, kale, chard
Strawberries	Collard greens

Note: Frozen fruits have been grown in the same way as fresh fruits, so check if your local store carries organic frozen fruit at a price that works for you.

OMG, GMO!

Genetically Modified Organisms are foods that are grown from seeds created in a laboratory. When food is a product of biotechnology instead of nature, its long-term effects on the body become questionable. Soy is one of the top GMO offenders, so that's why you should try to always choose an organic brand of soy milk. (Organic food cannot by law be GMO). There are only four vegetables and fruits grown from GMO seeds at present: some variations of zucchini, yellow crookneck squash, sweet corn, and papaya. The only one that may affect your juicing habit is GMO papaya from Hawaii.

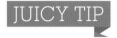

JUICY TIP

Produce stickers on supermarket foods can tell you at a glance if the fruit or vegetable is conventionally grown or organic. A 4-digit code is conventionally grown. A 5-digit code starting with a 9 signifies organic. A number 8 at the start means it's GMO. This labeling is optional however, so it's always better to look for an organic sign on the shelf itself.

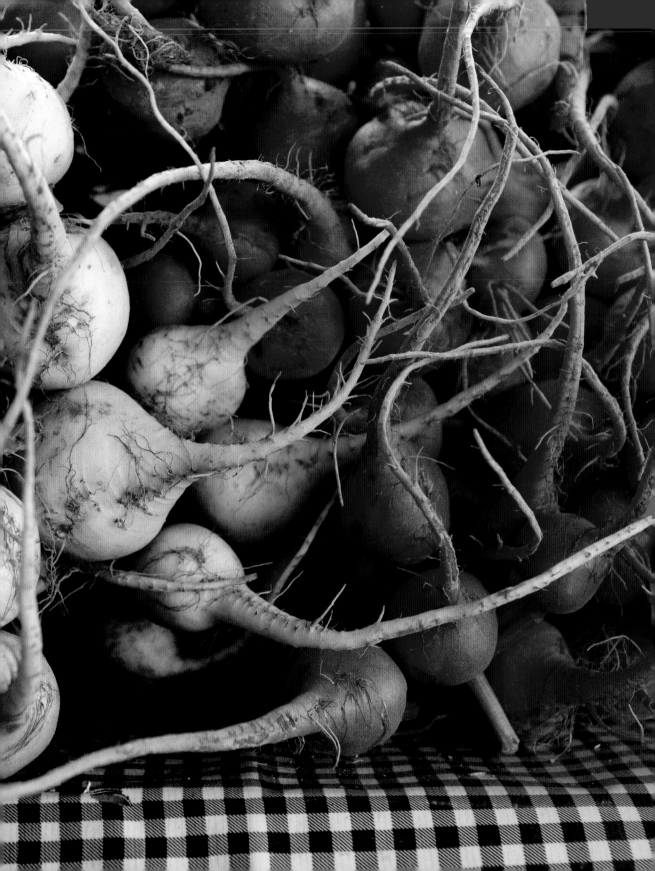

PREPPING
THE PRODUCE

Whatever your crunchy friends may tell you, washing all produce is very important. No matter where the fresh food comes from, dirt, germs, soil-born pathogens, human-carried pathogens, and exhaust fumes can all get on it, not to mention chemicals from pesticides, herbicides, and fungicides if it's not organic. Wash all produce well before using, swirling it well in your sink with your hands, and rinsing in fresh water. Scrub root vegetables with a special scrubbing brush under cold water. And wash all citrus fruits before cutting.

To ensure you've done the best job possible, add a tiny squirt of a bio-degradable produce wash to ensure contaminants like dirt and any petroleum-based chemicals on conventional produce, as well as applied waxes, are well removed. These tend to be made of food-grade cleansing agents. A little of this goes a long way: You can put some in a spray bottle of water and spritz it onto produce in the sink before rinsing well. Soak fragile berries and herbs in a very diluted solution of produce wash for a few minutes; then soak again in clean water. Of course, produce wash cannot remove the pesticides inside the produce, so it does not make it organic. But it helps. (In case it's not obvious, dish soap is not appropriate for this job!)

WASH YOUR WAY: THREE PRODUCE WASHES YOU CAN MAKE FROM YOUR PANTRY INGREDIENTS

Combine the following ingredients in a spray bottle: 1 tablespoon lemon juice + 1 tablespoon white vinegar + 1 cup water

OR

1 tablespoon baking soda +1 cup white vinegar + 1 cup water

OR

10 drops grapefruit seed extract + 1 cup white vinegar + 1 cup water

Spray on vegetables and fruit, let sit for 5 minutes, and rinse well under cold water using a scrub brush for hard vegetables and fruits.

Kitchen Wisdom: How to Get the Most from Your Precious Produce

Harder produce like apples, carrots, cucumbers, and pears can be washed in advance, then air dried on a towel and stored. More delicate leafy produce presents a problem: any remaining moisture will quicken the wilt in the fridge. Either salad-spin and leave to air dry extremely well before storing in the fridge, or wash as you need it.

Chopped vegetables will start to oxidize at the surface areas where they're cut. There's no science to show exactly how much this degrades the nutritional value. Keeping them whole until the last minute is preferred, but if chopping in advance helps you fit juicing into a busy day, go for it.

Drying the produce very well after washing and before storing is key. Kick it up a notch by storing your refrigerated produce in produce-saver, BPA-free plastic bags that use a natural mineral to help retain freshness. They are reusable many times over if you take care of them. Look for them in your health-food store. You can also invigorate wilting greens and herbs by storing them in jars of water in the fridge.

These fruits do not need refrigeration until they soften or you slice into them:

Apples

Apricots

Avocados

Melons

Nectarines

Peaches

Pears

Persimmons

Plums

Do not refrigerate the following:

Bananas (they will blacken)

Chiles

Garlic

Mangos

Pineapple

Sweet potatoes

Tomatoes

Root vegetables like carrots and beets do well with refrigeration, but also store pretty well in cool, dark places outside of the fridge if you take the leaves off. Herbs like parsley and cilantro can be kept on the counter with their stems in a glass of water.

Freshly juiced produce will start to oxidize the minute it's made. The best tip for saving juice for later is to put it in a jar that you can fill all the way to the top, so the juice touches the lid. This means it's not exposed to oxygen and won't oxidize further, retaining most nutrients. Put it in the fridge, because exposure to sunlight will also cause oxidization. Some experts think that 90 percent of the juice's value is retained this way if drunk within 12 to 24 hours. We don't recommend freezing your juice; it denatures it too much after all your good efforts. Smoothies typically endure a bit better in the fridge; again, store in an airtight container.

JUICY TIP

Glass jars are better than plastic for storing juice as plastic is permeable to oxygen. You can clean and save different size jars (think: salsa, nut butters, mustard, pickles) to have a range of sizes on hand, or use the American canning classic that's back in fashion with the foodie crowd: Mason jars.

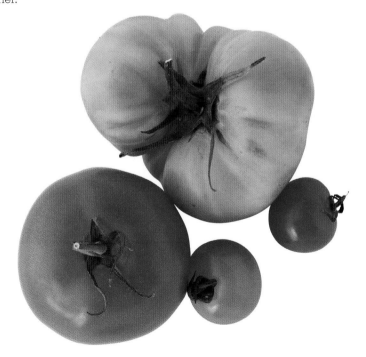

THE PULP PREDICAMENT

Cold-pressed juicers, like the Norwalk,
produce dry, jewel-toned pulp.

Every time you juice you make a lot of pulp. The vast majority of juicers trash this colorful mix in the name of time and convenience. Not so fast! It's full of good things for you and the earth. At Juice Generation, we compost every night and even put free pulp out for neighborhood gardeners, who come and fill baggies to take home to their plants. Consider keeping your juice pulp out of the landfill:

1 Use pulp in snack recipes. Juice pulp can be used to make flax crackers that are dehydrated in the oven on low or in a dehydrator. It's a gluten-free snack that is far cheaper than boxed crackers. A quick search online will reveal recipes for dehydrator crackers, as well as muffins and carrot cakes that use juice pulp. (Some juice blogs even post savory ideas like baked vegetable patties and throwing your pulp into vegetable stocks for soup.)

2 Compost it yourself: If you have a backyard, consider creating a compost pile in a corner for the increased amount of pulp and produce waste you'll be generating, and know your juice waste will go back into the garden. If you have a patio, a tumbler composter should fit easily and somewhat unobtrusively. If you're in an apartment with no outdoor space, an indoor compost contraption—aka a worm tower— is actually doable and delivers you a fertilizing "tea" that your house plants will adore. And if you live in a progressive city like San Francisco, Seattle, Boulder, or Portland, or in a neighborhood that is part of New York City's new green program, you're in business: Compost gets picked up by the city from your curb.

= A GREENER, = CLEANER KITCHEN

Juicing and blending require copious amounts of natural ingredients sourced from the earth—so when whipping up your favorite drinks it only seems right to bring some awareness to the environment from which they came. Just a few easy steps make a green drink even greener:

1 Turn the tap off! When washing produce, there's no need to keep water running for five minutes. Fill up your sink once, wash all your produce, then drain and fill a second time to rinse well.

2 When taking your drinks on the road, go for glass. Glass is free from harmful chemicals like BPA, phthalate, PVC, or polycarbonate that can leach into your beverage. Salvaged glass food jars make excellent to-go cups or look for a glass water bottle. If you prefer a less breakable vessel, get an insulated stainless steel thermos.

3 Next time you restock your under-sink supplies, try a natural cleaner for your countertops and reduce the toxic load of chemicals in your home.

4 Before reaching for a new pack of paper towels, stop! Chefs use washable kitchen towels in their kitchens—follow their lead and get a three-pack of cloths for cleanup and drying. (Lay wet vegetables on clean cloths to let them air-dry thoroughly before storing.)

5 Ditch the plastic baggies and shrink wrap: Buying your fruits and vegetables loose by the pound instead of prepacked is instant resource conservation. Take reusable sacks or recycled plastic bags of all sizes to the supermarket and farmers' market.

SIP TIPS

Believe it or not, the way you drink your juice or smoothie does matter!
Drink it at room temperature, not ice cold; this way it's easier to assimilate.
Try to resist gulping it down. Sip it slowly and swirl each sip a little in your
mouth so it mixes with saliva—this contains digestive enzymes that won't
otherwise be activated, as you're not chewing your food when you drink it.

It is good to drink fruit juices on an empty stomach as fruits digest very
quickly, and you don't want them to ferment in your stomach on top of
slower-digesting solid foods. Then wait 20 minutes or so before eating
anything solid. Vegetable juices also tend to give a more energizing effect
when consumed on an empty stomach. If drinking them as part of a meal,
pay attention to how your belly feels when food and juices combine. For
smoothies, it's a similar guideline: consuming them significantly before or
after a solid-food meal leads to better digestion

phase

LIGHT GREEN: BRIGHT AND REFRESHING

Give us five minutes of your morning; or maybe seven. Show up to your kitchen counter with your taste buds just the way they are and nothing but curiosity and a carrot—or ten—in hand. You've just stepped onto the Green Curve.

Nothing in this first phase of making liquid foods requires much preparation or many ingredients—and you're only going to dabble in the color green. This phase is all about small and reasonable steps. You don't even need to invest in a juicer in week one. A blender will do at first if you prefer to ease in conservatively.

Phase 1 is about simplicity and experimentation. You'll meet three key players who are set to become close compatriots on your juicing journey: celery, cucumber, and carrot. These humble vegetables, sometimes overlooked as no more than crudités, prove their preciousness when put through a juicer, because they produce so much liquid with such an array of benefits. They are "base" ingredients that form the foundation of your drink. Cukes and celery are also the two green vegetables that are the easiest to start with on your green journey: Because they're not ultranutrient dense, they don't have strong flavors, which makes them eminently palatable.

This first phase of juicing will also have you liquefying fruits that are positively bursting with goodness, like tart apple and vibrant orange and watermelon. And it offers a gentle introduction to the drinkable versions of two easy-to-find and nourishing leafy greens: kale and spinach. These foods offer a vast range of vitamins, minerals, and antioxidants as well as providing powerful health benefits—from blood sugar regulation to detoxification to improving your cardiovascular and circulatory systems.

Phase 1 also breaks down the smoothie into its simplest components and shows you how to whip one up with a variety of options.

These drinks skew a little on the sweet side. This is a deliberate tactic to lure your palate, not a long-term daily strategy. Be sure to try a range of the combinations in the days and weeks of Phase 1 and don't forget: Make sure a few of them contain spinach or kale.

THE TRADE-OUT: During Phase 1, set yourself a small challenge. Try to replace a midmorning or midafternoon pick-me-up drink with a juice or blended, and see how it makes you feel. After enjoying it, ask yourself: Do I have more energy or alertness? Do I still crave the caffeine top-up or energy drink? Could I do without it today? Don't make huge, hard goals if you don't want to—simply play with this new habit day by day and take a moment to see how it affects you. Use Phase 1 as a time to see how a fruit-and-veg boost can work for you.

Bonus: Phase 1 introduces you to satisfying and energizing drinks made without dairy. Limiting pasteurized dairy products throughout your day—like lattes, yogurt, and cheese—can be one of the most effective things to help you feel clearer, lighter, and brighter.

If this Trade-Out sounds deceptively simple, remember that in a world of rush-rush-rush and no-time-to-think, finding the time to stick something fresh in a juicer or blender is a little, sweet victory. You'll dial it up in the next phase as you learn the ropes.

Carrots, strawberries, Granny Smith apples, and spinach (for a touch of iron): It helps feed my soul and feed my cells and the carrots help me read the fine the print.

—**Katie Couric, journalist and broadcaster**

Hack That Juice! Two-in-one recipes make busy life a little easier. Throughout the book, we'll show you how to "hack" your juice, turning it into a smoothie with one added step.

PHASE 1
BUYING GUIDE

Your Green Curve goal in Phase 1 is to make juices or blended drinks with a 30 percent green factor—meaning at least some of them must contain greens. You can have them at any time of day that works for you. Try to incorporate both juices and blended drinks into your routine; the idea is to get familiar with both. Pick different combinations so that you've gotten acquainted with a range of ingredients and flavors and tried a spectrum by the end of this phase.

———

VEGETABLES

CUCUMBERS
CARROTS
CELERY
GINGER
BEETS
KALE
ROMAINE
PARSLEY
MINT
SPINACH

PANTRY

DATES
CINNAMON
ALMOND MILK
SOY MILK
COCONUT WATER
COCONUT MILK
PEANUT BUTTER
RAW ALMONDS

FRUIT

WATERMELON
ORANGES
PINEAPPLE
GRAPEFRUITS
APPLES
LEMONS
LIMES
BANANAS
FROZEN PEACHES
PEARS
MANGO
KIWIS
STRAWBERRIES

— PHASE 1 JUICES: —
CLASSIC COMBINATIONS

Sanya's
Gold Medal Greens

Race by the market stalls to fill your basket, and you'll have the fixings for a champion drink that delivers vegetables' benefits with a fruity finish.

1 cup spinach
1 cup parsley
½ small beet
2 medium apples
½ medium pear
4 medium carrots
Juice.

As an athlete, juicing is very important for me because I deplete my body with very intense training every day, and it's impossible to optimize my training without fueling my body with the best foods I can. Juicing makes it a lot easier to eat all the fruits and vegetables I need. The ingredients I use are also good for skin and hair health, inflammation, and coping with stress. I can tell the difference when I'm on a consistent juicing regimen: I am more alert, my recovery is at it's best, and I feel better.

—**Sanya Richards-Ross, four-time Olympic gold medalist in track and field**

Phase 1 introduces the essential ingredients of juicing. We show you the trios of easy ingredients that fill most juicing fan's fridges—things that harmonize well and that, even more important, deliver satisfying amounts of juice. They follow a flavor-combining pattern: They combine a neutral flavor that isn't too strong, plus a little sweet flavor and a little bold flavor that wouldn't work so well on its own. This achieves a balance in your cup.

The recipes give rough amounts of ingredients to make approximately 12 ounces of juice, but don't worry about being uber-exact. This is in-the-field training; if you get familiar with how much juice you tend to get from your produce, juicing becomes second nature. Unlike baking, which requires exact recipes to produce specific results, we believe that juicing falls under the "Italian grandma" style of food preparation; add a little of this, a little of that. Plus, there's some trial and error involved with discovering the perfect combinations of flavors. When adding ingredients to your juice or blended, think in terms of roughly packed cups, loose handfuls, or small pinches instead of exact measured ounces. Choose experimentation over precision. And have fun!

Not ready to splurge on a juicer yet? Try these combinations as blended drinks if your blender does a great job with hard produce, but add water or ice to make sure they blend. If your blender cannot handle hard produce, stick to the smoothies in this section the first week while you find a juicer that works for you, then start juicing in your second and third weeks.

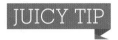

JUICY TIP

Start by juicing and blending things you already like to eat. You have to enjoy this to stick with it. In most recipes, the order of ingredients juiced is not written in stone. But there is a basic protocol: When juicing several fruits, juice the softest ones first, followed by the harder ones—this helps to push all their pulp through and extract maximum liquid. If using a centrifugal juicer, try rolling up your green leaves into cigar shapes to make them denser before pushing them through; follow with a harder vegetable or fruit.

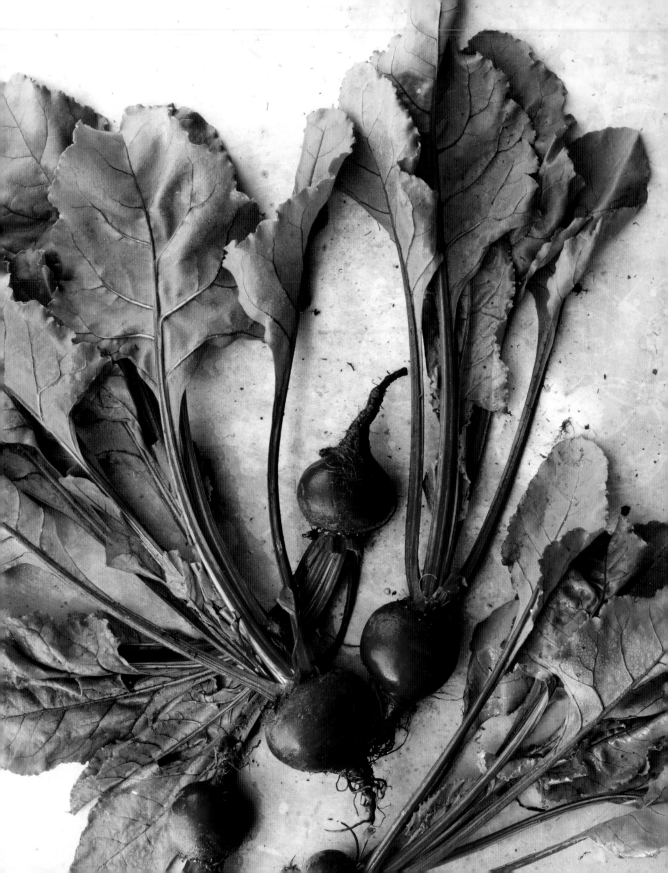

BEETS

Why We Love Beets

Beets are a welcome addition to any juice, adding palate-pleasing sweetness and equally satisfying health benefits. Beet juice has been found to lower blood pressure, purify the blood, and increase the production of glutathione, which helps the body eliminate environmental toxins. Scrub them well under running water, chop, and juice. (And keep the greens—you can juice them, too.)

CELERY

Why We Love Celery

1. It's one of the most hydrating foods we can put in our bodies.

2. Celery's incredible alkalizing effect helps to equalize the body's pH.

3. These stalks have special essential oils—you can probably smell them right away—that help regulate the nervous system and are very calming.

4. Celery supplies our cells with the soluble, live sodium they need to uptake nutrition and stay hydrated, which is why celery juice is a good rehydration drink for athletes.

Celery, Carrot, Spinach

2 stalks celery
4 medium carrots
1 cup spinach
Juice.

Hack That Juice! Blend with ½ a medium banana to make a smoothie.

Carrot, Beet, Spinach

4 medium carrots
½ small beet
1 cup spinach
Juice.

Carrot, Orange, Kale

4 medium carrots
1 medium orange, peeled
1 cup kale
Juice.

Hack That Juice! To turn your juice into a smoothie, pour into a blender and add ½ medium avocado.

JUICY TIP

Pick out carrots that are firm and smooth; ditch the ones that are cracked or molded. If you scrub the carrots well under water to remove all dirt, there's no need to peel. Chop the tops: Too many carrot greens can trigger your skin to burn in sunlight.

CARROTS
Why We Love Carrots

1. Carrot juice is sometimes called the golden juice of healing—it cleanses and restores the liver.

2. As a deep-soil root vegetable, carrots absorb an abundant array of minerals from the earth; they are especially rich in B vitamins and folate.

3. They have a surprising dark side: Early varieties of carrot were mostly purple and black. Our modern orange carrot stems from a mutant source that lacked those pigments.

4. When in a rush or in the mood for simplicity, carrot juice tastes terrific on its own.

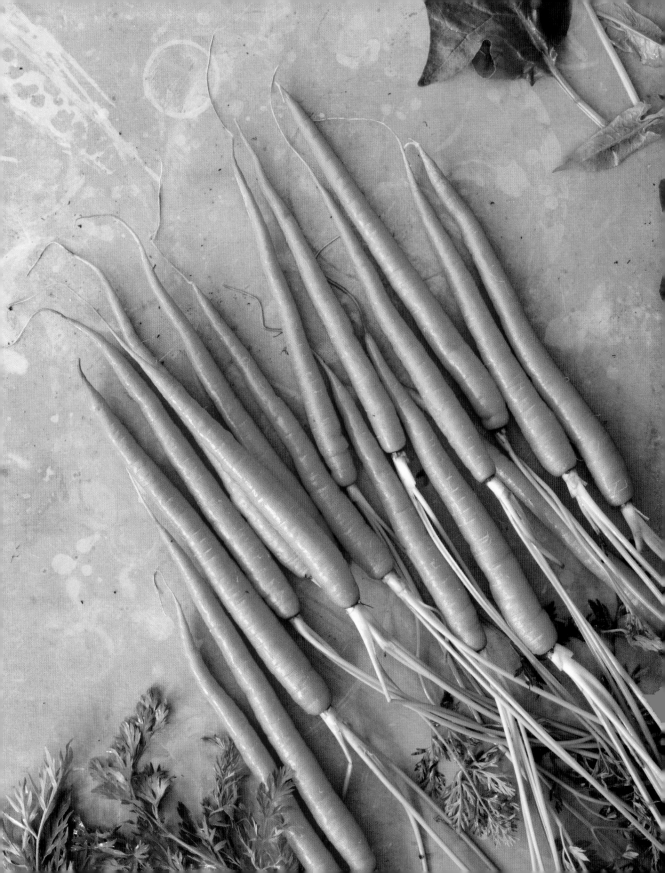

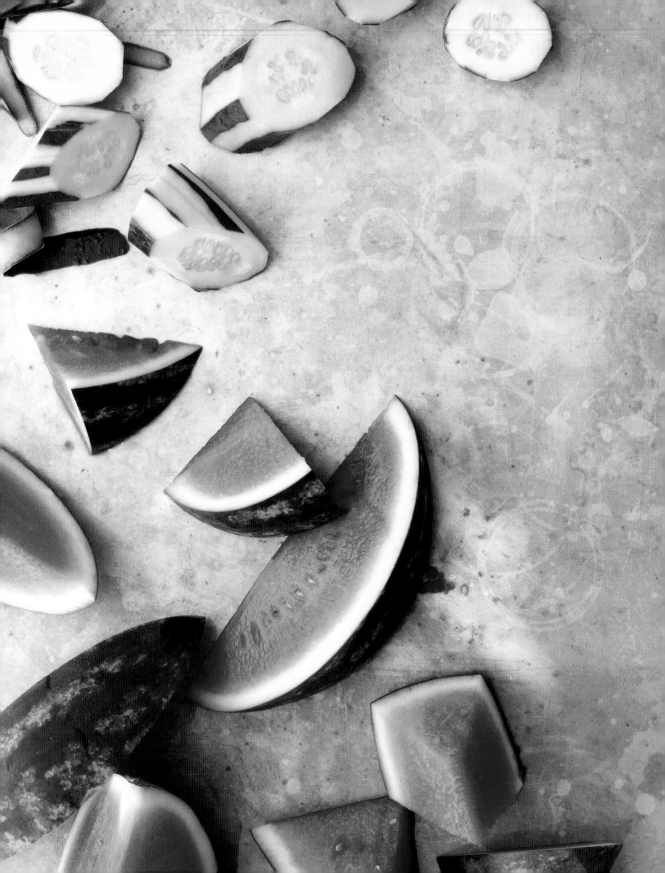

CUCUMBER 101

1. Put cucumbers in the juicer and watch the liquid flow—they are primarily made of water and deliver satisfying amounts of juice.

2. Their outer skin is a superb source of silica, a mineral that helps our connective tissue stay strong—and improves the complexion and skin health.

3. It plays well with others: Cucumber juice on its own doesn't have a whole lot of pep. But its neutral flavor makes it the perfect partner for almost everything else!

ORANGE 101

When juicing oranges, a juicer trumps a hand-held squeezer or citrus press because it puts the important nutrients from the pith into your drink. Wash and roughly peel your oranges, leaving as much white pith as possible on the fruit.

WATERMELON 101

Cooling, sweet, and quite low in sugar, watermelon offers a surprising twist: The rind has a concentration in minerals, antioxidants, and B vitamins as well the fruit's highest concentration of the amino acid citrulline, which supports healthy blood flow, supports detoxification, and refreshes fatigued muscles. If you can get organic watermelon and you wash it very well, juice part of the rind along with the flesh to get all the goodness. If it's not organic, it's safer to nix the rind.

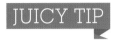

JUICY TIP

If your cucumbers are not organic, wash them very well. If they're waxed, be sure to peel them. Always pick cukes that are medium-to-dark green, not yellowed or aged.

Use blood oranges when available to up the ante on flavor, color, and wow factor.

Cucumber, Pineapple, Celery

½ medium cucumber

1 cup pineapple

3 stalks celery

Juice.

Watermelon, Orange, Cucumber

1 cup watermelon

1 medium orange, peeled

½ medium cucumber

Juice.

Watermelon, Pineapple, Lime

2 cups watermelon

1 cup pineapple

½ medium lime, peeled

Juice.

Cucumber, Watermelon, Lemon

½ medium cucumber

2 cups watermelon

½ medium lemon, peeled

Juice.

Celery, Pineapple, Ginger

6 stalks celery

1 cup pineapple

1 inch fresh gingerroot, peeled

Juice.

Orange, Apple, Spinach

2 medium oranges, peeled

1 medium apple

1 cup spinach

Juice.

Orange, Pineapple, Beet

3 medium oranges, peeled

1 cup pineapple

½ small beet

Juice.

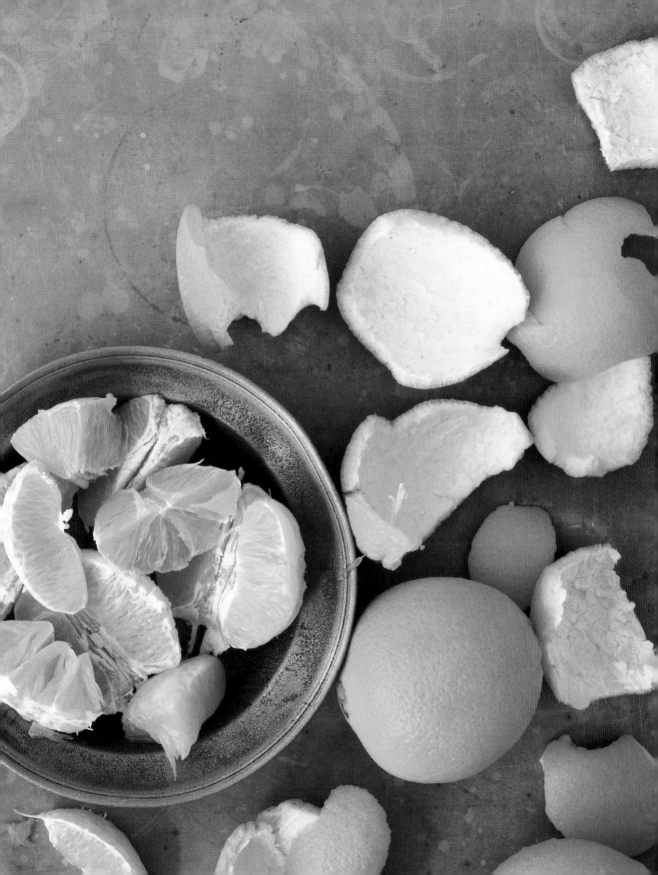

Green Apple, Ginger, Orange

1 medium green apple
1 inch fresh gingerroot, peeled
2 medium oranges, peeled
Juice.

Hack That Juice! Blend with ½ a medium avocado to make a smoothie.

THE G FACTOR: GINGER

This aromatic spice is one of the easiest ways to add a shot of spicy, warming flavor to your juices. But use a gentle hand—small amounts go a long way. The best way to spike your drink is to toss an inch-long knob into the juicer and judge how strong you like it. Look for firm, almost-hard ginger with unwrinkled skin. The thicker the skin, the stronger the flavor.

Combination Considerations: Some juicers (people, not machines) caution against combining fruits and vegetables in one drink, with the exceptions of green apples and carrots (they almost always get a pass to mix freely). The thinking is that the two food groups break down in the stomach in different ways, and this creates gas, bloating, and discomfort. Other juicers disagree, saying this is more of a philosophical idea than a physiological one, and it's not a hard and fast rule.

The best way is to get to know what works for you is to tune in to your own body's response. If you don't feel any gassy discomfort when mixing fruits and vegetables in your juices and smoothies, you are probably OK to continue. If you notice discomfort in your tummy, scale back to separate fruit-based drinks and vegetable-based drinks, with green apples and carrots available to both, and pay attention to the effect. If separating the two groups works better for your digestion, follow that path moving forward.

LEMONS
AND LIMES

Lemon and lime are a juicer's support crew. When thrown into juices, they add an energizing zing, have an alkalinizing effect—despite being citrus fruits—and mask bitter flavors, which makes them perfect companions for darker and more bitter green vegetables. Always have a stash of limes in your fruit bowl. If you overdo the darker greens like kale and get a too-bitter juice, another lime can help bring it back to balance.

FOR THE LOVE OF LEMONS

Morning juicing goes hand in hand with another easy habit: drinking hot water and lemon on waking. It especially helps if you're pledging to decrease caffeine. As you make your morning juice, sip on the lemon water and enjoy its uplifting effects. It floods your body with alkaline fluid, which is helpful as the body becomes more acidic overnight through digesting and detoxifying. It dissolves mucus and helps to flush the liver, helps you absorb minerals better, and encourages the formation of bile in the gallbladder, which helps to break down fat. It also helps to stimulate the bowels to move in the morning. If you enjoy the taste, drink this simple mix throughout the day—warm or cool.

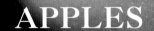

APPLES

Don't overlook the humble apple. Taken for granted as an everyday fruit, the humble apple is a shining star in raw juices, which showcase its popping flavor. At Juice Generation, we get our apples from a historic New York State orchard that grows more than 30 different varieties, and we think exploring the spectrum of apple varietals is a journey in itself. Tart, green apples are the primary, low-sugar choice for mixing with vegetables to make green drinks; red varieties like Fujis have an irresistible, pear-like flavor for a sweeter drink. And there are many, many more to try.

It doesn't take much effort to extract the specialness of an apple. A simple combo of one or two ingredients is enough. Try varying red and green apples to learn their flavors and sweet-tart effects.

I am relatively new to juicing and I can honestly say the difference I feel is HUGE. Every morning on set I have my "green" drink, which is spinach, kale, cucumber, lemon, celery, green apple. Sometimes I'll add beets, and if I'm under the weather I'll add ginger. I'm not a big green vegetable eater, so the juice really has filled a huge void in my diet, and I feel stronger for it.

—**Debra Messing, actor**

Debra's Green Elixir

The neutral greens of celery and cucumber plus the sweetness of apple and beet make this admirably green juice balanced enough to be completely inviting, not intimidating.

3 leaves kale
1 cup spinach
1 medium apple
5 stalks celery
¼ medium cucumber
½ small beet
½ medium lemon, peeled
Juice.

Tropical Lust

Pineapple is high in bromelain, an enzyme that helps the body digest proteins and reduce inflammation. Eating—or drinking—fresh pineapple is not only a gustatory delight, it can help reduce swelling and pain from injuries.

2 cups watermelon
¾ cup pineapple
1 medium apple
1 inch fresh gingerroot, peeled
Juice.

Red Delicious

Orange and carrot add depth and color to red apple juice plus another gift: a good dose of vitamin C and beta-carotene.

1½ medium red apples
5 medium carrots
1 medium orange, peeled
Juice.

Apple Zing

Ginger adds a spicy kick while delivering anti-inflammatory benefits and soothing digestive distress like nausea.

3 medium apples
1 inch fresh gingerroot, peeled
½ medium lemon, peeled
Juice.

Apple Mint Smoothie

Proof that fruits, vegetables, and a blender can be best friends. In this drink, that minty multitasker peppermint offers an uplifting hit that is high in potassium, iron, and calcium as well as vitamins A, C, and E.

1 bunch fresh parsley
¼ medium cucumber
½ medium apple
½ medium frozen banana
1 sprig fresh mint
1 cup filtered water
Blend.

Daily Detox

Diversify from the typical carrot juice with the supremely hydrating addition of cucumber and a twist of apple for maximum thirst-quenching refreshment.

5 medium carrots
¼ medium cucumber
1 medium apple
1 inch fresh gingerroot, peeled
½ medium lemon, peeled
Juice.

JUICY TIP

Want to try making an apple "juice" in your high-speed blender? Add some water to help it liquefy, and expect a thicker puree. Just remember to remove the woody stem.

Apple Picking

Look for apples that are firm and well-colored—more color means the apple was picked when it was more mature, which means it will have more flavor and longer lasting power. An apple that's soft to the touch is overripe. Farmers' markets often have "visually distressed" boxes of organic apples that are a little dinged up but great for juicing.

Juice Smarts: Apples are a rich source of pectin, a gel-forming soluble fiber that helps your intestines draw out toxins and excrete waste, as well as helping to reduce cholesterol.

PINK, WHITE, WHAT'S RIGHT?

Ruby red (also called pink) grapefruit has far more vitamin A than the white-yellow varieties, as well as antioxidants that help lower blood sugar levels and lycopene, which has antitumor properties. The pink fruits also tend to taste considerably sweeter. But both kinds have their fans: Do a taste test and see what you like best. Whichever you choose, pick fruits that are firm, feel heavy for their size, and have no green color showing in the peel.

THINK MINT

Try a touch of mint to add refreshing flavor to sweet and tart fruit juices, coconut blends, and lighter green smoothies. This easy-to-grow herb is soothing on digestion and has some antiviral benefits—but as with many delicate leaves, you may find it juices better in a masticating juicer or high-speed blender than a centrifugal juicer.

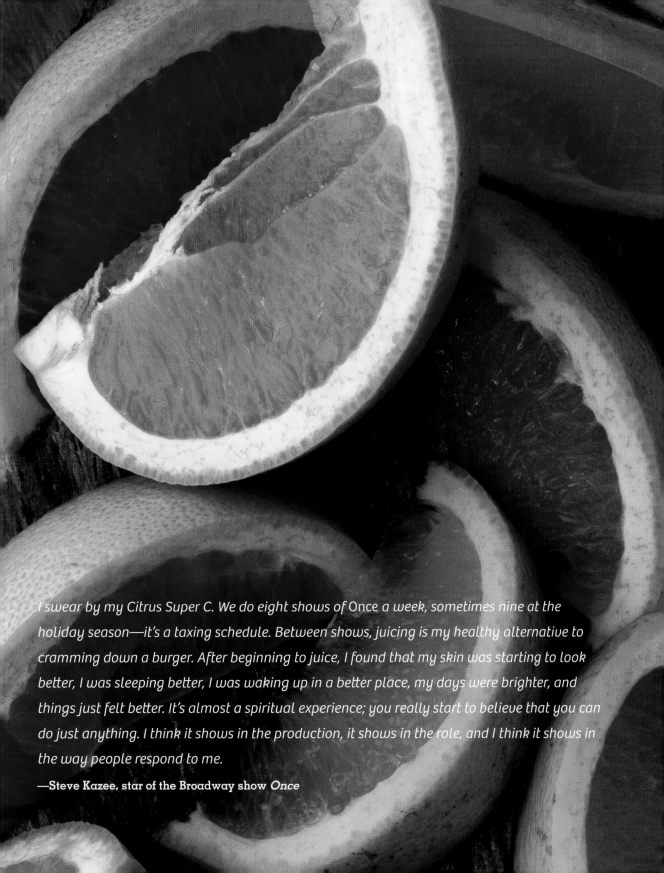

I swear by my Citrus Super C. We do eight shows of Once *a week, sometimes nine at the holiday season—it's a taxing schedule. Between shows, juicing is my healthy alternative to cramming down a burger. After beginning to juice, I found that my skin was starting to look better, I was sleeping better, I was waking up in a better place, my days were brighter, and things just felt better. It's almost a spiritual experience; you really start to believe that you can do just anything. I think it shows in the production, it shows in the role, and I think it shows in the way people respond to me.*

—Steve Kazee, star of the Broadway show *Once*

GRAPEFRUIT
Tart 'n' Tangy: Energizing Grapefruit Combos

Grapefruit's bold flavor is complemented by bright additions like mint and ginger. Add more or less as you see fit!

Grapefruit is your energizing wake-up call. Ditch the idea that grapefruit is breakfast for retirees (you know: half a grapefruit with a side of prunes and a cherry on top). This morning glory is better seen as *classic*. And for good reason: Grapefruit has powerful properties to aid the kidney, liver, and gallbladder and, taken first thing in the morning on an empty stomach, you'll feel its tingle of cleansing, refreshing energy. It's also got a special extra twist: It stimulates the liver to go into fat-burning mode.

Make grapefruit part of your breakfast of champions with a few simple ingredient combos. It's shockingly easy to draw out every sparkling facet of grapefruit—and discover why its Latin name is *Citrus paradisi*.

It's important to always peel your grapefruit before juicing, because the peel is toxic if ingested. Conventionally grown grapefruit will also have a lot of pesticides on its peel. But leave as much of the white pith on as possible—it's a rich source of phytonutrients.

Citrus Super C

¾ cup pineapple
½ medium grapefruit, peeled
2 medium oranges, peeled
1 sprig mint
Juice.

Grapefruit Refreshmint

2 medium grapefruits, peeled
1 sprig mint
Juice.

Grapefruit Moon

1½ medium grapefruits, peeled
½ medium pear
1 inch fresh gingerroot, peeled
Juice.

Grapefruit Zinger

2 medium grapefruits, peeled
1 inch fresh gingerroot, peeled
Juice.

The Grateful Grapefruit Juice

Can you blend your grapefruit? Absolutely: it's a fabulous way to keep the fiber intact, too. The better your blender, the more smooth and silky your drink will be.

2 medium grapefruits, peeled
½ cup peach
½ medium banana
1 tablespoon raw agave
½ cup ice
Blend.

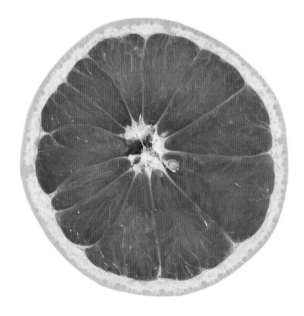

Juice Smarts: Grapefruits contain an enzyme that interacts with some prescription medications, including certain cholesterol-reducing, psychiatric, and impotence drugs—often dangerously enhancing their effects. If you're on medication, check with your doctor for contraindications before getting a serious grapefruit juice habit.

Juice Smarts: If you juice or blend a lot of cruciferous vegetables like kale, make sure your diet is well supplied with iodine, which is found in kelp and other seaweeds. Adding ½ to 1 teaspoon of powdered kelp to a smoothie every so often is a superb way to do this. You can also use iodized salt, multivitamins, or iodine supplements. You need adequate amounts of iodine because consuming large amounts of raw cruciferous vegetables may interfere with thyroid hormone action in some people by blocking the utilization of iodine. If your dietary iodine levels are adequate, it should all balance out. If you have a known thyroid issue, consult with your health practitioner about the amount of raw kale that is wise for you. In Phase 2, we'll tell you why it's smart for everyone to rotate their greens.

KALE

At the Juice Generation stores, we go through crates of kale each day. We're huge fans of this humble vegetable—despite its intimidating, so-green-it's-almost-black appearance—because it scores number one on the vegetable scale of most micronutrients per calorie. Many juice gurus say that kale has such a strong flavor—and bold effect on the body—that it is for expert juicers only. But we beg to differ: If you ease in moderately, it's never too soon to start using the leaf that packs the biggest nutritional punch. Juiced on its own, kale has a way-too-bold taste. But if you combine kale with the right ingredients and in the right balanced amounts, you can enjoy superb nutritional benefits *and* satisfying flavor. The sweeter combos here help to downplay its naturally bitter (read: good for you) taste. Don't try to drink supersize glasses of kale juice—it's concentrated nutrition and you only need a little to benefit.

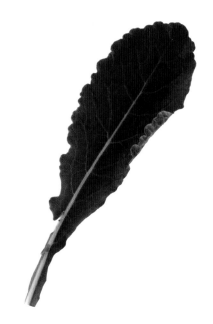

WHY KALE IS KING

1. It's available year-round because it's hardy in cool weather and a survivor in hot weather.

2. It's durable and lasts for some time in the fridge.

3. There is an array of varieties, from the slightly bitter curly kale, to the dark green, earthy dinosaur (also called lacinto) kale, to the purple-stalked Russian kale, and more. Try whatever looks freshest and most appealing, notice any differences in taste and juice volume, and rotate your choices through several varietals for maximum nutrition.

4. It's a cruciferous vegetable, part of the same family as cabbage, collards, broccoli, and cauliflower (also called the brassica family), which contain unique sulfur-containing compounds that provide a spectrum of anticancer benefits. Kale supercharges the natural protective mechanisms of our cells, and helps prevent deposits of plaque inside blood vessels. It's a health and longevity miracle food!

I am obsessed with any and all green juices. Cut spinach, kale, or Swiss chard with a little lemon or apple, and you can't even tell that you are drinking something ridiculously good for you. Making healthy food choices and preparing them takes a great deal of time, often time that I don't have. Juicing takes the work out of the equation and frees me from thinking about food so I can concentrate on other things. I can't think of anything that makes me feel as good and is as easy to do.

—Michelle Williams, actor

JUICY TIP

When juicing kale, the whole leaf can go through the juicer. When blending kale in a smoothie, roughly tear the leaves off the thick stems, then compost or trash the stems.

Michelle's Leafy Green Goodness

Three kinds of green leaves deliver potent nutrition in an easy-to-drink blend of fresh apple. Use tart green apples to lower the sugar content if you like.

3 leaves kale
1 cup spinach
2 leaves Swiss chard
4 medium apples
½ medium lemon, peeled
Juice.

TropiKale: Kale + Pineapple

Dark, green kale is surprisingly refreshing when combined with clean, sweet pineapple. And the two are nutritional dynamos, creating a juice brimming with calcium, antioxidants, and vitamins K and C.

1 cup kale
2 cups pineapple
Juice.

Hail to Kale

A Juice Generation bestseller, this classic recipe has helped thousands of juicers fall unexpectedly in love with the wonder that is kale.

1 cup kale
1 cup watermelon
1 medium apple
½ medium lemon, peeled
Juice.

Emerald + Orange: Kale + Carrot

Sometimes the simplest combos are all you need. 2 powerful ingredients with two vibrant colors.

1 cup kale
5 medium carrots
Juice.

Leaves & Roots: Kale + Carrot + Beet

A blend of above-ground and below-ground vegetables treats your body—and your taste buds—well.

1 cup kale
4 medium carrots
½ small beet
Juice.

— PHASE 1 SMOOTHIES: —
PURE SIMPLICITY

Back in about the late 80s, the smoothie burst on the scene in a riot of sherbet and fruit juice. Thick, goopy, frosty, and oh-so-sugary, these tropical and vivid-hued concoctions weren't exactly paradigms of health. They were jazzy, tangy, exciting fun foods—*a new twist on the milkshake!*—that were often found alongside the smoothie's best friend, frozen yogurt. We could sort of feel good about them, because of all the fruits. But with that sugar rush-and-crash, and probably a fair dose of colorings and flavorings, they sure left us feeling a little worse for wear.

Today, we're in the middle of a smoothie revolution! Sherbet is out—and vegetables, nut milks, exotic fruits, performance protein powders, superfoods, and medicinal herbs are definitely in. The landscape of blended drinks has totally evolved. We're waking up to the pressing need for more fiber, and much more enzyme action, in our diets and connecting the dots between deficiencies and disease. A new appreciation for green smoothies has millions chucking spinach and parsley into their blenders with crusading zeal, eating pounds more greens than ever before.

It's funny how the passion for upping the ante with new ingredients can sometimes make us forget that a blended drink doesn't have to be complicated to be good. A few ripe and tasty things combined with a good-quality base will deliver a satisfying snack that sneaks lots of vibrant nutrition into our diets with absolutely minimal effort. Just wash, blitz, and go.

The smoothies in this section show you—or remind you—just how easy it can be. Pick a base liquid; select a fruit or two; try sneaking in some greens; and if you feel you need it, add a touch of extra sweet in the form of dates to blend the flavors together. A little sweetness can help downplay the vegetable factor for those taking a first foray into green drinks.

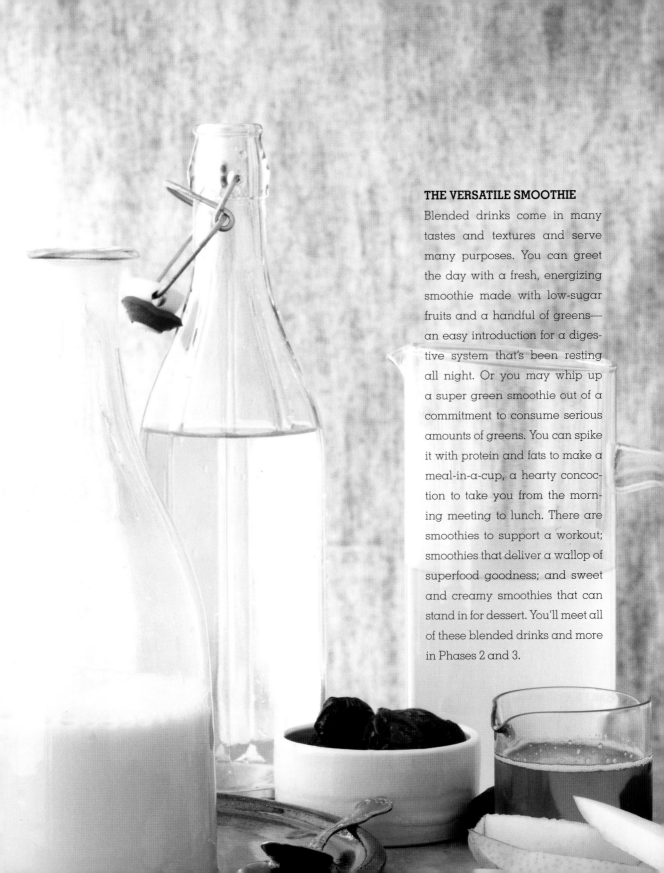

THE VERSATILE SMOOTHIE

Blended drinks come in many tastes and textures and serve many purposes. You can greet the day with a fresh, energizing smoothie made with low-sugar fruits and a handful of greens—an easy introduction for a digestive system that's been resting all night. Or you may whip up a super green smoothie out of a commitment to consume serious amounts of greens. You can spike it with protein and fats to make a meal-in-a-cup, a hearty concoction to take you from the morning meeting to lunch. There are smoothies to support a workout; smoothies that deliver a wallop of superfood goodness; and sweet and creamy smoothies that can stand in for dessert. You'll meet all of these blended drinks and more in Phases 2 and 3.

THE ESSENTIAL COMPONENTS

It's simple. First, find a base liquid. Next, add fruits and vegetables. Then blend. These juicing prerequisites will make you a seasoned smoothie-maker in no time.

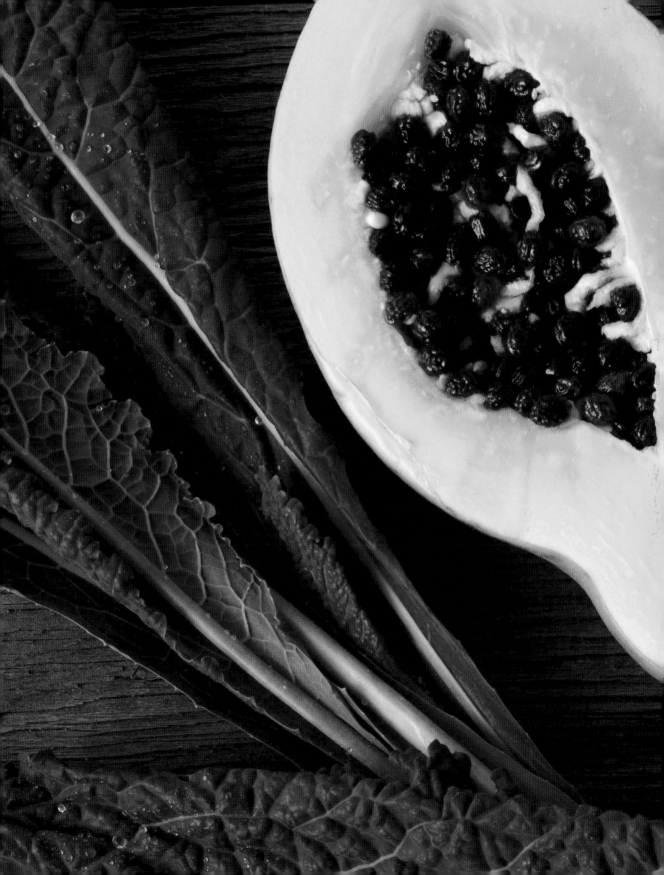

1 FIND YOUR BASE

The base is the liquid carrier for whatever fruits and vegetables you choose to use. Without it, you'll get a pureed mush—or possibly paralyze your blender. You can play with a spectrum of liquids here to get different kinds of drinks:

Water A totally valid base liquid for many a smoothie, especially those bursting with fruits and greens. It won't add any flavor, so make sure everything else in the drink is popping with taste. Filtered water is ideal. Bottled water, due to its impact on the environment, is less so.

Fruit juice Tangy and tasty, but don't get hooked on big quantities of store-bought juice every day (see Juice Imposters, page 37). You only need to use fruit juice in moderation—and a good trick is to add splashes of bold-flavored juices, along with water, into your mix (like pomegranate, acaí, and berry-cherry blends).

Juice your own When possible, we like to juice our own apple, orange, and watermelon and then add to smoothies. It takes a few minutes more, but it's the freshest and most nutritious way to put nature's bounty into your cup, and the taste is incomparable.

Coconut water Boxed coconut water is a big business these days as everyone discovers its refreshing effect, life-supporting electrolytes, and lower-fructose composition. We much prefer drinking from fresh young coconuts—introduced in Phase 2—but packaged varieties are time-saving and can work well in smoothies. There's a huge variety in flavor; the best you'll get (at a higher cost) are the new "100% raw" coconut waters that are pressure-pasteurized (rather than heat-pasteurized). Canned ones may have added sugar or preservatives—but not always. Read the labels.

Nut milk The easy way to add a richer, creamier texture, a decent amount of protein, and a little fat to your drink is with a nut milk. You'll find a great amount of choices on supermarket shelves, from nut, seed, legume, and grain bases. Look for almond, soy, hemp, oat, rice, flax, hazelnut, and coconut milks—and more. Many offer good nutrients and are a fine dairy substitute, but the convenient boxed versions come with a downside: Most contain some added cane juice for sweetening and additives like preservatives, and they are pasteurized, not fresh made. When nut milks are sickly sweet, they overwhelm your fresh fruits and vegetables. It's best to look for unsweetened, unflavored versions (you can use natural sweeteners to adjust the final taste) and with soy milk in particular, make sure it's organic. Stick with us through Phase 3 and we'll show you the absolute best way to get your nut milk on—make it yourself!

Juice Smarts: A seaweed-derived ingredient called carrageenan is often used in boxed soy and nut milks as a thickening agent. Some people find it aggravates gastro-intestinal problems; if these liquids irritate your stomach, seek brands without it.

2 FOCUS ON FLAVOR : SMOOTHIE-CENTRIC FRUITS

Some fruits taste better than others when whirred into a blended drink. Our top smoothie-tastic ingredients include berries (think: blueberries, raspberries, strawberries, blackberries, acaí berries, and even the superfood goji berry). Berries work wonders in a blended drink; they're low in sugar, but high in flavor and color—practically bursting with healing antioxidants. They work well with nut milks and with less dense liquids like coconut water. When they're not in season frozen organic is a good stand-in. Peaches and tropical fruits like mango, pineapple, and papaya are also delectable—and enzyme- and vitamin-packed—additions to any smoothie.

Bananas and avocado—also a fruit—are a smoothie's best friends because their high volume of soluble fiber means they blend brilliantly, integrating all the ingredients into a creamy, even texture. Fruits like pears, papaya, mango, strawberries, and kiwis also have high amounts of soluble fiber. Make a smoothie without these natural thickeners—especially if you are using water or coconut water instead of nut milk—and your smoothie may be chunky or stringy, or separate slightly.

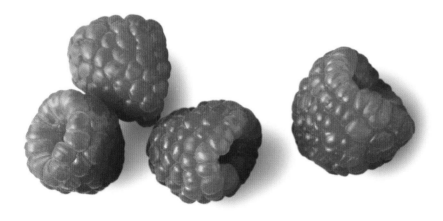

3 GREEN UP YOUR CUP

Almost any kind of smoothie can be easily greened by tossing some leaves into the blender. Spinach is the classic smoothie green as it has a mild flavor that mixes beautifully with other fruits. Kale, the nutritional powerhouse, has a stronger flavor that can be balanced with bright fruits like berries and pineapple. Swiss chard, romaine lettuce, bok choy, and collard greens are also excellent additions and you can even experiment with savory flavors of beet greens and spicy mustard greens in vegetable-only smoothies. Start slowly as you get to know your greens—in Phase 1 the focus is on spinach and kale. Add a small handful to your blender before committing to a deeper green experience.

4 THE FROST FACTOR

Adding ice to your smoothie is a personal choice. On the upside, it can transform a simple smoothie into a decadent, milkshake-like experience, enhancing its flavor and texture. Those watching their weight appreciate how it fills out the drink without adding extra calories. On the downside, ice can make your blended drink too frosty, which can make it harder to drink and—many healers say—be a shock to the digestion, slowing it down. If you're using frozen fruit, you don't need ice. (And if frozen fruit in your smoothie is too teeth-chattering, splash hot water on top to melt it slightly before adding the other ingredients.)

5 SWEETENING THE DEAL

If the ingredients in your smoothie don't quite satisfy your palate and you need it a touch sweeter, use a natural sweetening ingredient that is as unprocessed as possible and experiment with the amounts you need. Aim to decrease the amount of sweet gradually as you get used to enjoying the full flavor spectrum and already-occurring sweetness of your drink.

All very sweet things have lots of calories—there's no getting around that. But some contain higher amounts of fructose—the supersweet kind of sugar molecule that can have the most damaging impact on the body and that gets stored quickly as fat if you eat more than a moderate amount. Choosing what sweetener to use involves balancing your taste preference with an awareness of fructose amounts—and of course, over the long term, adapting your palate so you need only a touch of sweet to be satisfied. Some of our favorite sweeteners include:

Dates These sumptuous dried fruits are not only outrageously delicious, they contain an array of antioxidants, trace minerals, and both soluble and insoluble fiber to add more oomph to your hit of sweet. Two or three medium-size dates in a smoothie or homemade nut milk will more than satisfy your desire (and even one may be enough). You can find fresh dates in most markets; look for plump dates with smooth and unwrinkled skins. They can last for several months when refrigerated in a tightly sealed container. Dried dates can last for up to a year in the fridge (they can be "replumped" with warm water if they dry out). Soaked raisins, figs, and prunes also add sweetness that kids especially will like—an even healthier option is to use the soaking water itself and save the fruits for something else.

Raw honey One of nature's most potent gifts, raw, unfiltered honey is beloved by raw foodies and healers alike because it is so high in healing enzymes, has a great trace mineral content and phenomenal healing compounds like propolis, and is lower in fructose than other natural sweeteners. Unlike conventional honey, raw or unpasteurized honey hasn't been heated and filtered to make perfect-looking golden syrup, and it is free of the questionable things in the cheapest honey products (which may contain high fructose corn syrup, illegal additives from overseas, and zero beneficial pollen).

It's also one of the easiest "wild foods" to acquire—it's now available at stores like Trader Joe's—and when you get your honey from farmers' markets, you help support local beekeepers who are crusading to save our utterly essential bee population—ensuring we can continue to grow food in the future! A dash of raw honey is like putting preventive medicine in your food. Start with 1 tablespoon in your smoothie and adjust downward from there as your palate adjusts.

Raw agave Made from the agave plant—the source of tequila—agave syrup is a low glycemic sweetener that, if processed properly, can have a moderate fructose level, a lower caloric content than table sugar, and inulin, a prebiotic fiber proven to help the absorption of certain nutrients. Look for raw, organic agave that can claim a fructose level of under 50 percent (which is sugar's fructose level). Some agave brands are highly processed and contain a much higher percentage—from 70 to 90 percent, which is as bad as high fructose corn syrup.

Coconut palm sugar The new kid on the block, coconut palm sugar is made from dried and crystallized sap from the coconut tree. It's being embraced for its wonderfully rich, caramel flavor—similar to brown sugar—and its gentler effect on blood sugar than regular sugar. You get a shot of vitamins, minerals, and phytonutrients, and sensitive types might notice they don't get a jittery sugar rush from adding it to their drinks.

What we don't recommend: artificial sweeteners like aspartame and sucralose, which are made of chemicals and connected to a host of health problems from cancer to neurological issues and everyday mind fog and pain.

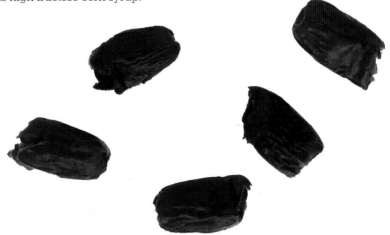

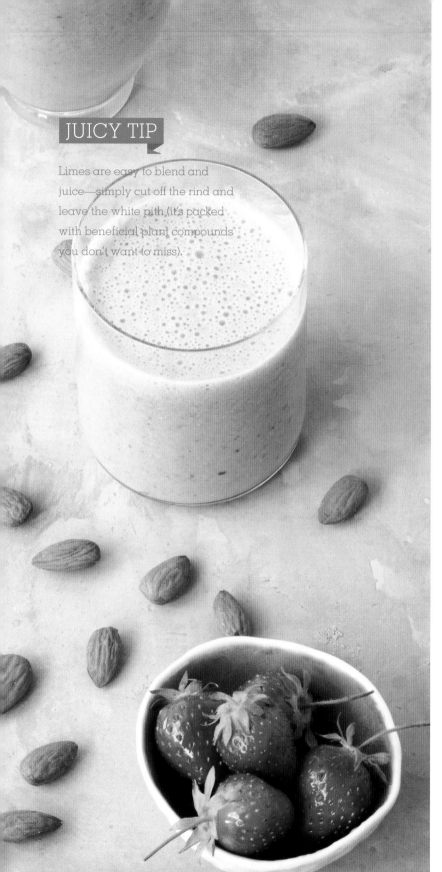

JUICY TIP

Limes are easy to blend and juice—simply cut off the rind and leave the white pith (it's packed with beneficial plant compounds you don't want to miss).

Peaches and Greens

Creamy almond milk combined with sweet peaches and dates makes this smoothie a dessert-worthy affair. Peaches are high in the antioxidant chlorogenic acid, which slows the aging process and prevents chronic disease.

1 cup spinach
½ cup peaches
½ medium frozen banana
1 cup almond milk
3 dates, pitted
Blend.

Clean Green

This superbly refreshing smoothie spikes dark-green kale with bright-green lime, an ingredient that balances kale's bitterness beautifully

1½ cups kale
¼ cup cucumber
1 medium apple
1 medium lime, peeled
1 cup filtered water
Blend.

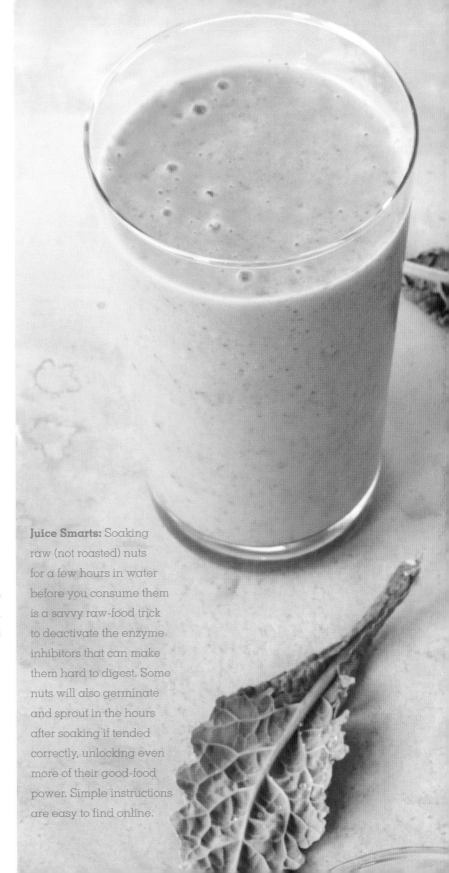

Tropical Greens

Don't overlook the furry brown kiwi. This little fruit is jammed with nourishment, offering 16 percent of the RDA for fiber as well as folate, vitamins C and E, and minerals including calcium, magnesium, potassium, and zinc.

1 cup spinach
½ cup pineapple
½ cup mango
1 medium kiwi, peeled
1 cup almond milk
½ cup ice
Blend.

Nuts for Greens

A handful of raw almonds makes a smoothie into a meal. They add protein, omega-3 and omega-6 fatty acids, plus lots of fiber.

1 cup spinach
¼ cup raw almonds
1 cup almond milk
½ cup strawberries
½ cup blueberries
½ medium frozen banana
Blend.

Juice Smarts: Soaking raw (not roasted) nuts for a few hours in water before you consume them is a savvy raw-food trick to deactivate the enzyme inhibitors that can make them hard to digest. Some nuts will also germinate and sprout in the hours after soaking if tended correctly, unlocking even more of their good-food power. Simple instructions are easy to find online.

NOT GOT MILK

Juicing was the beginning of my deeper understanding of nutrition. The great feeling and positive physical results I got from early experiments with "juice fasting" made a big impression on me and made me start paying more serious attention to the connections between what I was eating and my health. The older I get, the more aware I am of how unhealthy most of what passes for food in our culture has become. Personally I'm trying to eat simpler and cleaner and stick to a whole-food, plant-based diet. I'm pushing myself to go as green as I can with juicing and keep the fruits to a more modest percentage. I feel better and it keeps my energy more even.

—Edward Norton, actor

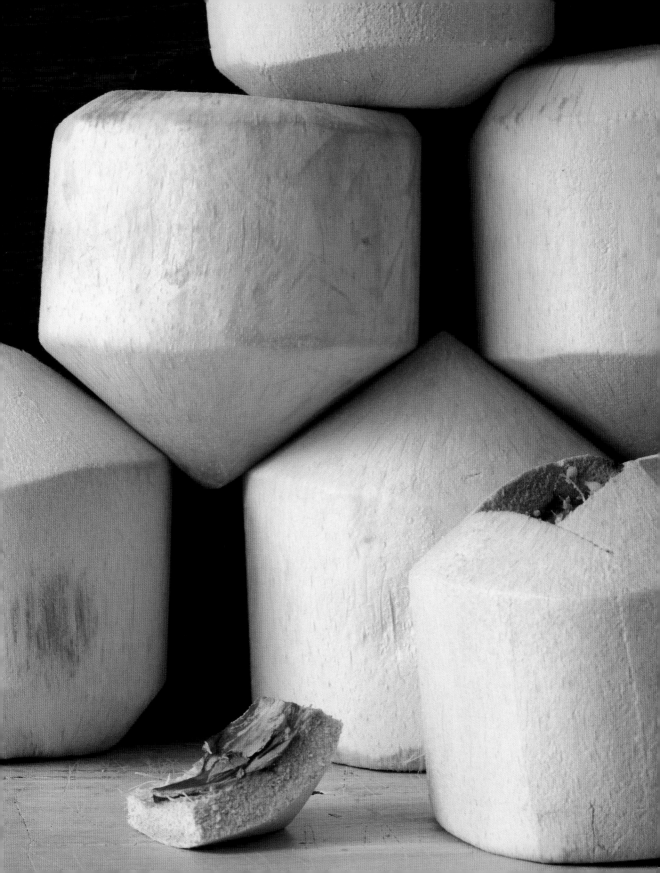

Juice Smarts: Soy milk has its fans and its detractors: Some worry that its naturally occurring phytonutrients have estrogenic effects on women (promoting, and preventing healing of, breast cancer). Other reputable heath gurus disagree, saying it's a great milk substitute with phytonutrients we need. If you choose to use soy milk, use a product bearing the green USDA Certified Organic seal; soy beans are heavily treated with pesticides and are often GMO; many are often shipped in from overseas where "organic" standards may be questionable. And if you're not sure, drink soy moderately: With so many choices on the shelf, it's easy to rotate your nondairy milks (just like you'll rotate your greens!).

The smoothies on the Green Curve are free of dairy—there's no yogurt to thicken and enrich them—because on the Green Curve, we want to give you a chance to do a Trade-Out and bring your consumption of dairy products down, to see how it feels for you.

We're not saying dairy in all its forms is terrible for everyone. But there's no denying that dairy is one of the most inflammatory foods in our modern diet, and it's connected to all sorts of gut issues, persistent skin symptoms, mucus formation, and much more, due to both the sugars and the proteins milk contains. And, unless it's organic, dairy can be full of growth hormones and antibiotics; two things you do *not* want in your—and your children's—bodies.

Our recipes offer you an opportunity to nix some of the milk products in your diet and instead discover the enriching textures of nut milks and coconut meat. Don't worry about getting your calcium. You'll get lots of it from plant foods like almonds, kale, oranges, collard greens, and spinach on the Green Curve, which are also wonderfully alkalinizing.

Cocoverde

Whizz together two fruits, plus greens, plus banana and you've got a classic green smoothie: almost instantaneous, and equally pleasurable to the eyes and the palate. Here, nutrient dense kale and tropical mango—high in vitamins A, C, and D as well as beta-carotene—mingle beautifully in a coconut water base that's tasty and hydrating.

1 cup kale
½ cup mango
½ medium frozen banana
1 cup fresh coconut water
Blend.

Optional: Add 1 teaspoon cinnamon for a special twist.

Perfectly Pear

Fusing three shades of green into one pale-hued smoothie, this concoction is irresistible to look at—and drink. Pear adds a delicate, sweet flavor—plus lots of soluble fiber—while romaine lettuce contributes its wonderfully mild-flavored leaves.

1 cup spinach
2 leaves romaine
1 medium pear
½ medium frozen banana
1 medium lemon, peeled
1 cup filtered water
Blend.

JUICY TIP

Cinnamon—a spice once considered more valuable than gold—is still revered today for its ability to help lower blood sugar levels.

Hack That Smoothie! Make any smoothie instantly more filling with a generous spoonful or two of fats like avocado, nut butter, or chia seeds. This is especially great for kids, who'll like the tangy flavors of these entry-level blended drinks, but need a little more substance to keep them going. It's wise to let the chia seeds "plump out" in liquid for ten minutes before drinking so they add hydration to the body effectively.

BANANA 2.0

Shake off the childhood memory of the squished banana at the bottom of your brown bag lunch. This versatile, superbly nutritious fruit elevates an everyday juice into a milkshake-worthy smoothie with just the flip of a blender switch. Bananas add sweetness, body, and a silky smooth feel to blended drinks (they're how healthy beverages masquerade as luscious treats). And they play well with others. Blend bananas with almond milk and cacao nibs for a smoothie that drinks like a dessert; mix banana with coconut water, mango, and greens for a vibrant tropical beverage, and whiz banana with peanut butter and any dairy milk substitute for a creamy, protein-packed delight.

———

BANANAS: WHAT DON'T THEY DO?

Bananas are nature's energy shot. Packed with healthy carbohydrates and potassium, they are ideal for a pre- or post-workout boost, helping to restore the body's electrolyte balance. Bananas are famous for their potassium for good reason: The mineral helps to maintain healthy blood pressure and protect against arteriosclerosis. They also contain pectin, a soluble fiber, which helps to ease constipation, while the tryptophan in the fruit is converted to serotonin, which helps us feel happier. Bananas build strong bones by preventing calcium loss and they are a natural antacid, providing relief from acid reflux and heartburn.

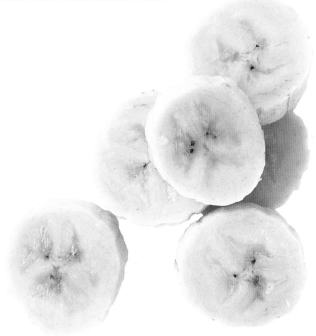

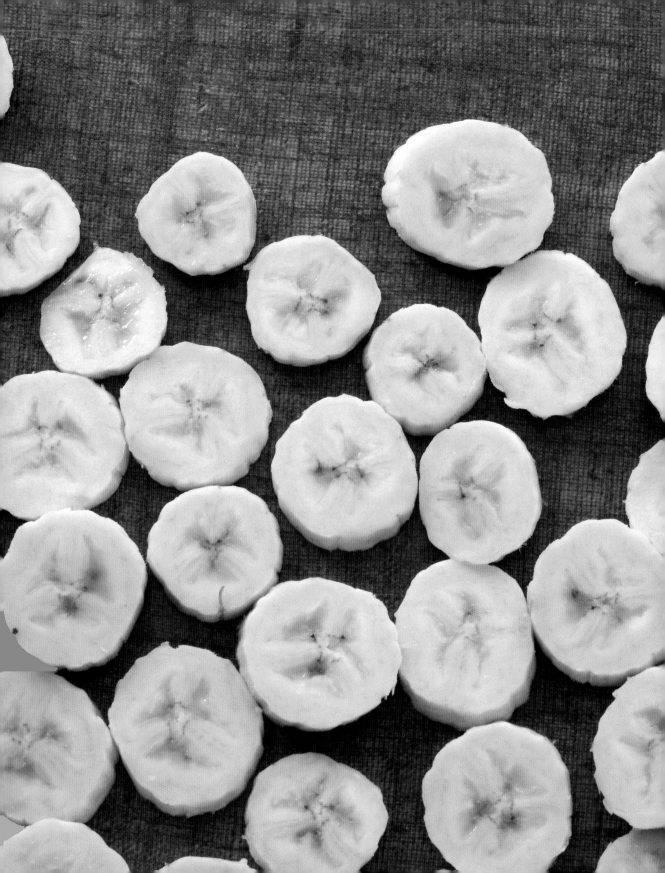

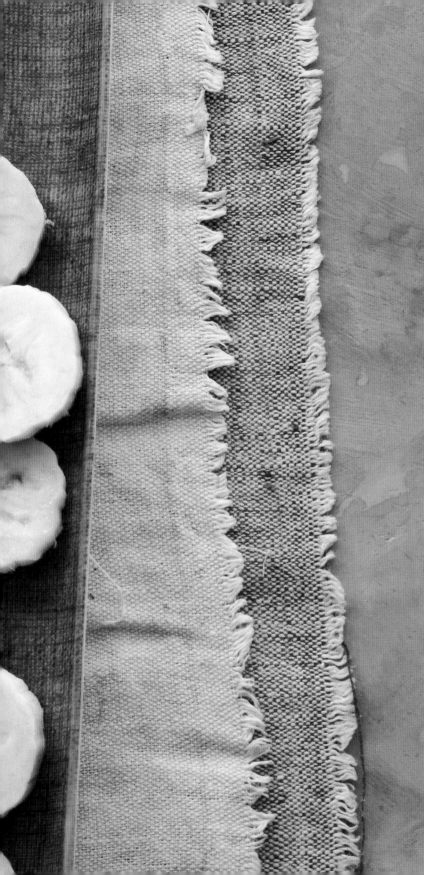

Smooth Strawberry

Juicing your apples before blending this smoothie is one extra step that pays off. Use green apples for a tarter drink and red ones for a sweeter blend.

1 cup fresh apple juice
½ cup strawberries
½ medium banana
sweetener to taste
½ cup ice
Blend.

PB Split

When you need a little more substance to get you through the day, a smoothie boosted with nut butter, nut milk, and coconut milk will fuel you with fat, the body's favorite source of energy, without a ton of sugar.

2 tablespoons peanut butter
1 medium frozen banana
1 cup almond milk
¼ cup frozen coconut milk
1 tablespoon raw agave
½ cup ice
Blend.

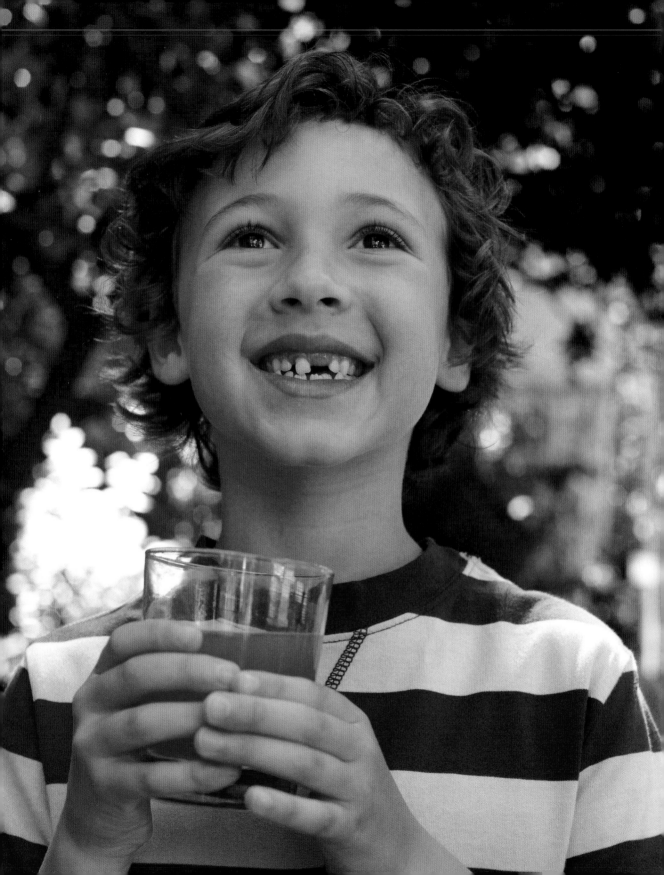

— WHIZ KIDS —

For kids, blending tends to work better than juicing initially, because thicker, creamier drinks are more palatable and more entertaining to drink. Transitioning to juices can be just as enjoyable, however. Most kids will shy away from green in their drinks at first, but get sneaky and add a handful of kale or spinach to fruity concoctions when they're not looking, or come clean and let your kids see that sometimes it's easy—and tasty—being green.

Drinking juices is extremely satisfying: I feel like I'm being rewarded with every sip, especially with the green juices, and watching my children drink all those greens is the greatest feeling, knowing they are consuming all the right nutrients. I sleep better at night knowing that all the goodness from the veggies and fruits has gone directly into our systems. There's too much messing with food these days, so the purity of juice makes it the nectar of the gods!

—Naomi Watts, actor

Kid-Approved Juice Combos

Apple, pear, spinach

Apple, pear, celery, cucumber

Apple, carrot, romaine

Pineapple, kale, apple

Carrot, orange

Beets, tangy citrus

Combos with coconut water

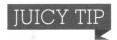

JUICY TIP

Deep red beet pulp makes a colorful mix-in for healthy muffins and treats that kids find especially irresistible.

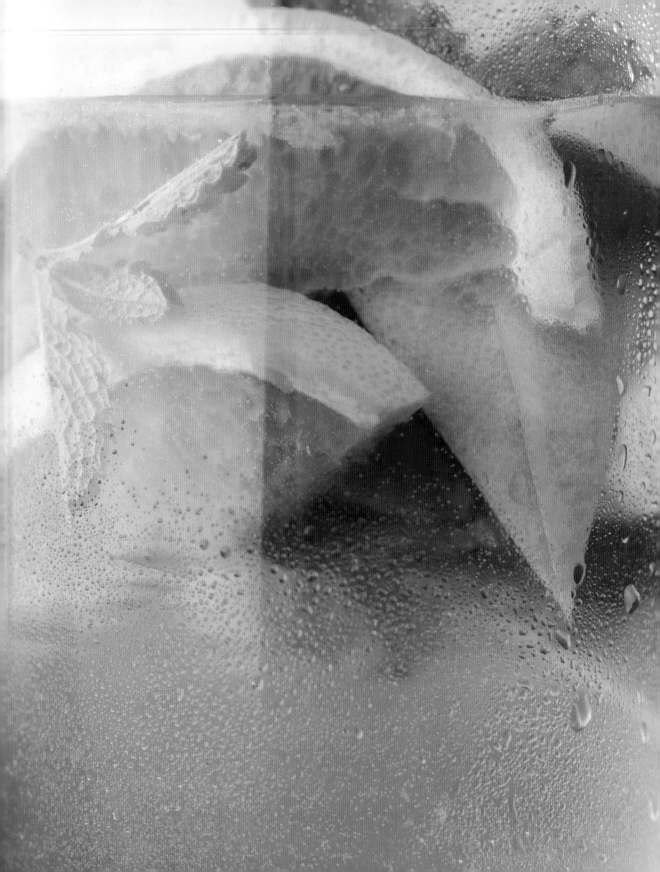

AGUA FRESCA

Fruit and herb-infused water is one of the easiest natural beverages to make at home. They're fun for kids to make and create a beautiful-looking drink to serve your friends.

Try using some of the ingredients you already have on hand to make these simple, but restaurant-worthy, drinks. There's lots of room for experimentation here; get creative with ingredients that you feel may go well together and let the inspiration flow.

METHOD: Place your fruits and vegetables in a pitcher or glass mason jar and lightly mash with the end of a wooden spoon. Amounts can be fairly rough—fill the bottom of your vessel and throw in a small handful of herbs. (You can always add more herbs next time if necessary.)

Gently bruise your herbs or spices like mint and ginger on a cutting board first, so they release their flavor, then add to the mix.

Fill your container with still or sparkling water, sealing it if using sparkling water, and let sit in the fridge for at least two hours. Strain before serving. Use within approximately two days.

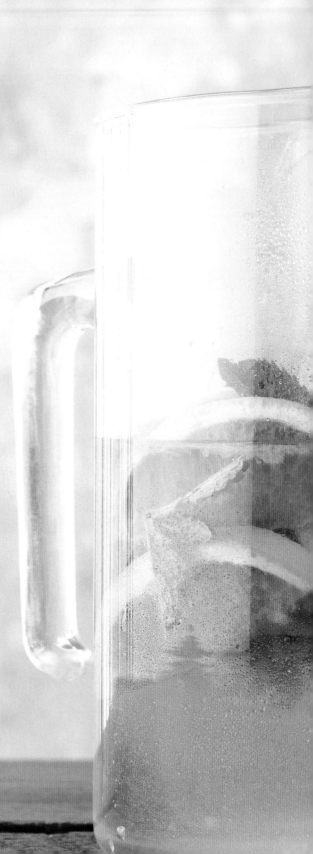

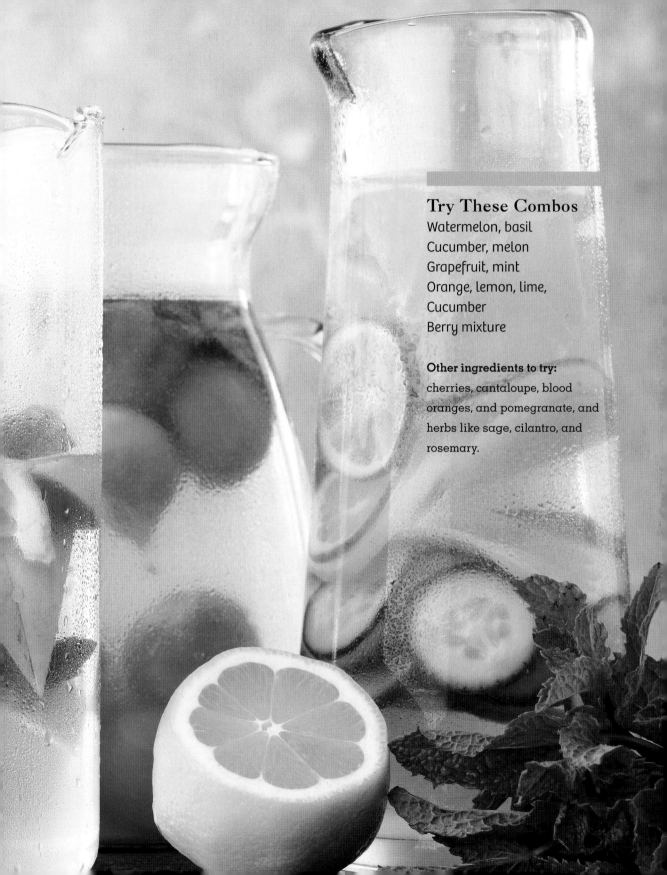

Try These Combos
Watermelon, basil
Cucumber, melon
Grapefruit, mint
Orange, lemon, lime,
Cucumber
Berry mixture

Other ingredients to try:
cherries, cantaloupe, blood
oranges, and pomegranate, and
herbs like sage, cilantro, and
rosemary.

phase

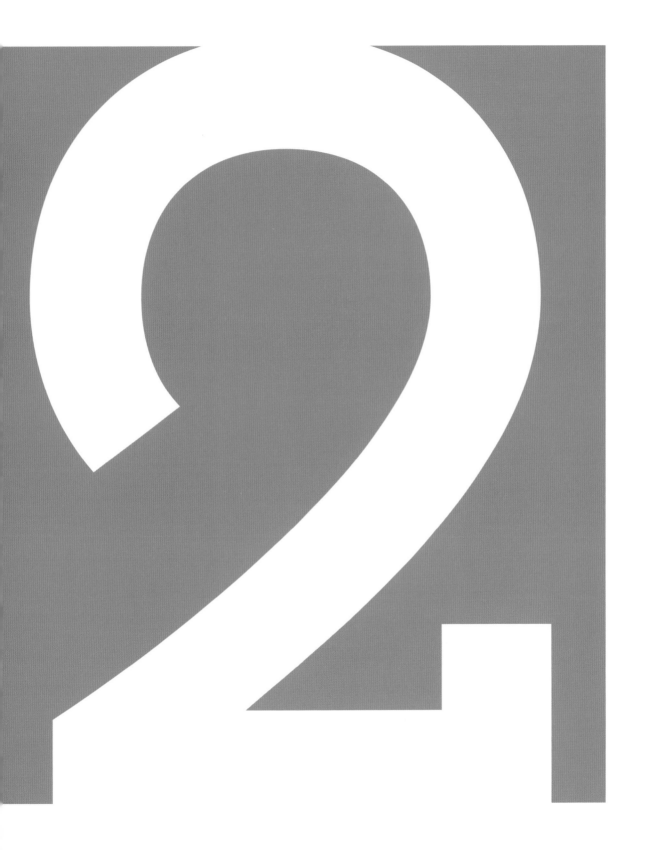

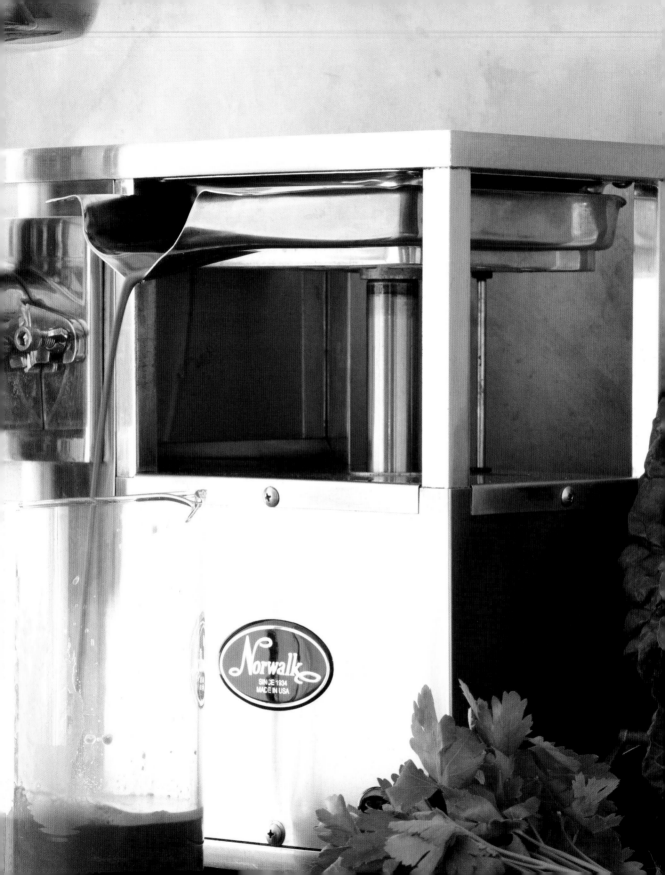

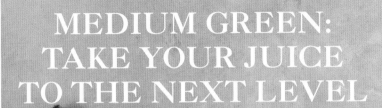

MEDIUM GREEN: TAKE YOUR JUICE TO THE NEXT LEVEL

I am ruled by my juicer. Anything green that's not nailed down ends up being juiced. Kale, spinach, a little green apple, and we are good to go. It's also an easy way to get a salad in my six-year-old and one-year-old. If my wife is right and you are what you eat, I'd rather be lean and green than hot and beefy.

—Jason Bateman, actor

On the second part of the Green Curve, you explore a wider array of flavors and colors, including more shades of green. This phase is about expanding your palate and broadening your scope from sweeter tastes to those with a more savory slant, and incorporating many new shades of green in your glass. There are tasty treats galore in store: You'll crack open coconuts, get friendly with hemp (one of nature's humble superstars, a secret weapon of nutrition), blitz an array of unexpected vegetables in your juicer, and discover the joy of flavor-bursting açaí bowls. You'll also discover smoothies with a little more substance that are just the ticket as a heartier snack or perhaps a recovery meal in a cup after a workout.

While it's good to follow your body's wisdom and use ingredients you find appealing, it's also important to stretch a little, and try things you've never even heard of or thought to use—these surprises can often turn out to be the best!

Plan to stay on Phase 2 for three weeks to try a wide range of the recipes and get to know a diversity of new ingredients at a realistic pace. But if you would rather go at your own speed and flip ahead for new recipes sooner, you can do that, too.

THE TRADE-OUT: Phase 2 is an opportunity to drop packaged, sugary, and salty snack foods from your diet and replace them with nourishing drinks. Cookies, muffins, pastries, and pretzels may be an occasional or a frequent fallback habit, but what about switching them out for a fresh juice or smoothie instead? And how about the chips, nachos, bread roll, or French fries that keep showing up with your lunch—what if you had a green drink half an hour before your meal, to cut the craving for those things? If you have a family, how about giving your child a thermos of cool, green smoothie for a brain- and body-fueling school snack?

These switches may require lifestyle adjustments—like taking your juice or smoothie on the road in a cooler bag or stashing a bottle in the fridge at work. But a little thinking ahead lets you reap rewards. Cravings for sugar, baked goods, fake flavors, and candy highs get a chance to fade from focus and you can begin to detect, and desire, new types of fresh, nutrient-rich foods.

Bonus: Goodbye, gluten. We're waking up to the ways that gluten—the protein found in wheat, barley, and rye and used as a hidden filler in many modern foods—can disrupt our physical and mental well-being through intolerances, allergies, and in extreme cases, an auto-immune response. Gluten's ubiquity can make it a challenging thing to remove from your daily diet. Fresh juices and smoothies made filling with fats and protein can take the place of wheat-filled breakfast foods like cereal, toast, and pastries, and they offer great new alternatives to snacks that may have been irritating your system for years, undetected. (This includes oat-based breakfast and snack foods that, unless marked "gluten-free," often contain the gluten protein.)

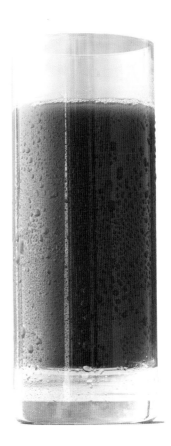

PHASE 2
BUYING GUIDE

Your Green Curve goal in Phase 2 is to make five drinks in a week with at least 50 percent containing significant greens. During this phase, aim to make at least five drinks a week—which may be each weekday to get in a rhythm, or three weekdays plus two weekend days, when you have the most time to get creative. Pick and choose the juices and smoothies you want to make as you see fit—you can pull from Phase 1 if you need—but now try to ensure at least half of them contain a good handful of leafy greens. Make them at any time of day that fits in your schedule.

VEGETABLES

DAIKON RADISH
WATERCRESS
SWEET POTATO
SWISS CHARD
AVOCADO

PANTRY

FLAX OIL
COCONUT OIL
ALMOND BUTTER
HEMP MILK
PROTEIN POWDER
HEMP SEEDS
HEMP GRANOLA
RAW CACAO NIBS

FRUIT

BLUEBERRIES
FROZEN ACEROLA CHERRIES
RASPBERRIES
YOUNG COCONUTS
FROZEN ACAI BERRIES
DRIED GOJI BERRIES

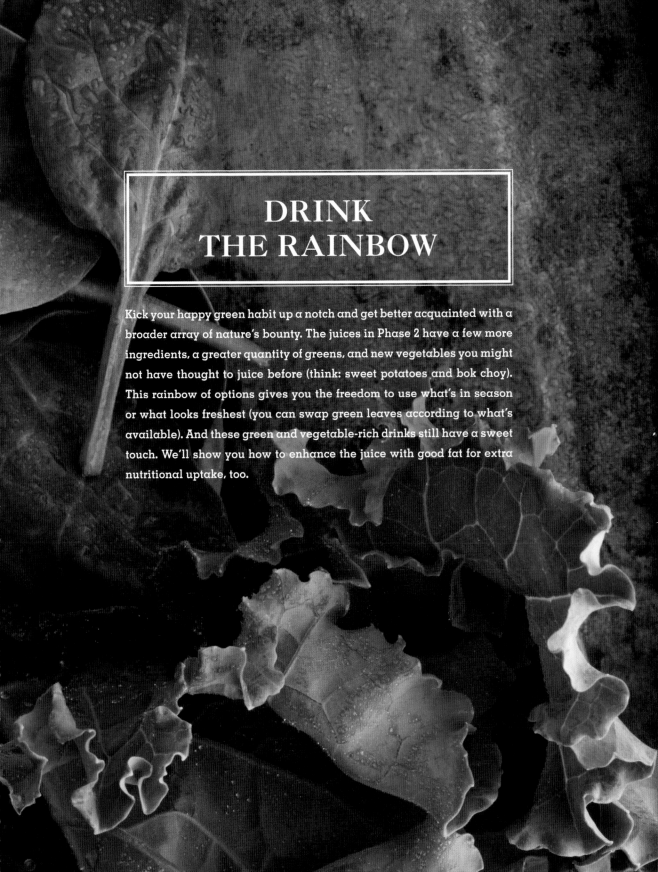

DRINK THE RAINBOW

Kick your happy green habit up a notch and get better acquainted with a broader array of nature's bounty. The juices in Phase 2 have a few more ingredients, a greater quantity of greens, and new vegetables you might not have thought to juice before (think: sweet potatoes and bok choy). This rainbow of options gives you the freedom to use what's in season or what looks freshest (you can swap green leaves according to what's available). And these green and vegetable-rich drinks still have a sweet touch. We'll show you how to enhance the juice with good fat for extra nutritional uptake, too.

I juice a wide array of fruits and vegetables according to what I feel my body needs at that time, from spinach to beets to my favorite combination: carrots, green apple, and ginger. This is what I drink when I find I need more energy in my work: It's a great pick-me-up. In summer, I love fresh watermelon juice—it's a sweet treat that's healthy. What I've learned is that our bodies tell us what we need. It's up to us to listen and follow that guidance.

—Hilary Swank, actor

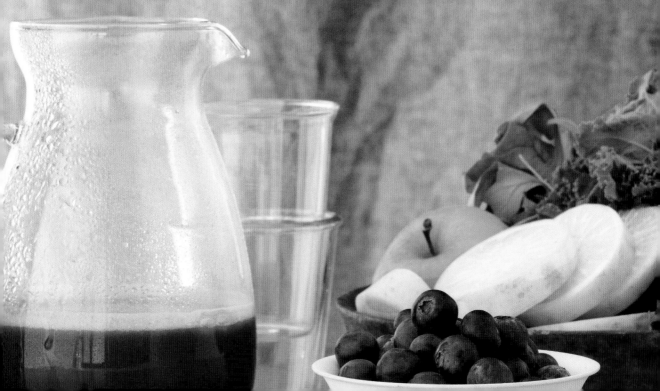

Very Veggie

Sweet potato as juice? You bet. This pumpkin-colored tuber is not only a surprising—and easily sourced—ingredient with an appealing flavor, it also helps you get your glow on. The carotenoids in orange-colored vegetables like carrot and sweet potato have such beneficial effect on skin, they have a scientifically validated "attraction factor"—meaning that warm glow you naturally acquire makes others rate you as more attractive.

1 cup kale
1 cup spinach
1 cup parsley
¼ medium sweet potato, peeled
¼ medium cucumber
4 medium carrots
3 stalks celery
Juice.

Get Ur Green On

It's never been easier to go green. Here, nutrient-packed kale and spinach are sweetened with apple and pineapple and brightened by mint. Young juicers tend to fall for this tasty green number.

1 cup kale
1 cup spinach
½ cup pineapple
2 medium green apples
1 sprig mint
Juice.

Hack That Juice! Blend in ½ cup fresh coconut meat to make a smoothie.

SupaDupa Greens

Juice Generation's
Number One Selling Drink

Get ready for graduate level greens. This fortifying brew is big on green veggies and light on fruit, making it satisfyingly savory. Cucumber refreshes and lemon harmonizes, creating an uplifting, energizing drink.

2 cups kale
1 cup spinach
1 cup parsley
2 leaves romaine
3 stalks celery
1 medium green apple
¼ medium cucumber
¼ medium lemon, peeled
Juice.

Hack That Juice! Blend in ½ medium avocado to make a smoothie.

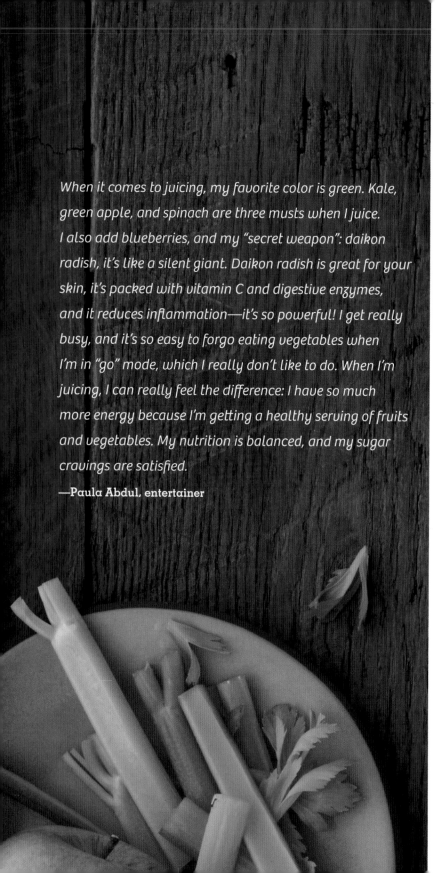

When it comes to juicing, my favorite color is green. Kale, green apple, and spinach are three musts when I juice. I also add blueberries, and my "secret weapon": daikon radish, it's like a silent giant. Daikon radish is great for your skin, it's packed with vitamin C and digestive enzymes, and it reduces inflammation—it's so powerful! I get really busy, and it's so easy to forgo eating vegetables when I'm in "go" mode, which I really don't like to do. When I'm juicing, I can really feel the difference: I have so much more energy because I'm getting a healthy serving of fruits and vegetables. My nutrition is balanced, and my sugar cravings are satisfied.

—Paula Abdul, entertainer

Paula's Daikon Blues

Looking like a white icicle and pleasantly mild in flavor, daikon's crisp, cool properties make it tons of fun to juice. A hit of blueberries adds a second surprising twist.

½ small daikon radish
1 cup kale
1 cup spinach
2 medium green apples
Juice.

Hack That Juice! Blend in ½ cup blueberries.

Sweet Greens

Explore nature's bounty with the addition of two power greens: watercress and parsley. Peppery watercress contains iron, iodine, vitamins A, C, and E, antioxidants, and folate, while parsley is so much more than a mere garnish. The herb is bursting with vitamins plus iron, calcium, magnesium, potassium, and zinc.

1 cup spinach
1 cup kale
½ cup parsley
½ cup watercress
3 medium apples
Juice.

Hack That Juice! Blend in ½ medium banana to make a smoothie.

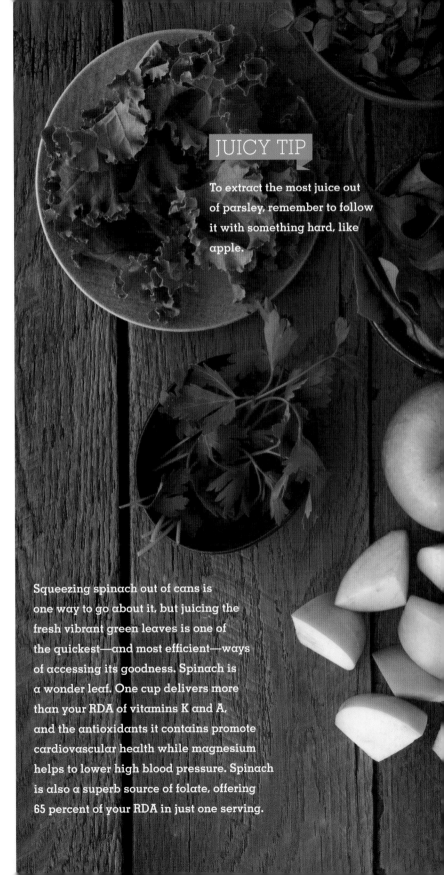

JUICY TIP

To extract the most juice out of parsley, remember to follow it with something hard, like apple.

Squeezing spinach out of cans is one way to go about it, but juicing the fresh vibrant green leaves is one of the quickest—and most efficient—ways of accessing its goodness. Spinach is a wonder leaf. One cup delivers more than your RDA of vitamins K and A, and the antioxidants it contains promote cardiovascular health while magnesium helps to lower high blood pressure. Spinach is also a superb source of folate, offering 65 percent of your RDA in just one serving.

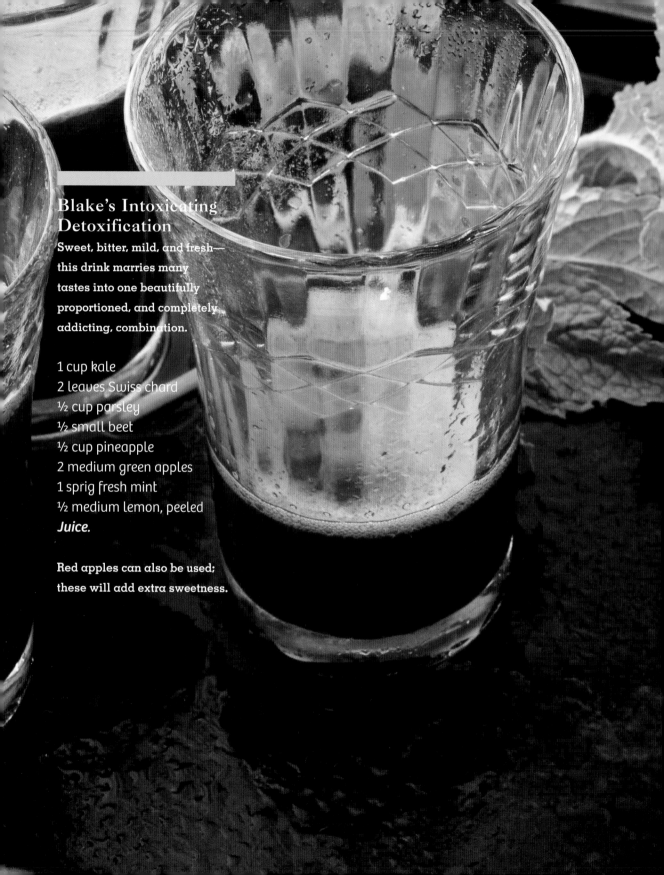

Blake's Intoxicating Detoxification

Sweet, bitter, mild, and fresh—
this drink marries many
tastes into one beautifully
proportioned, and completely
addicting, combination.

1 cup kale
2 leaves Swiss chard
½ cup parsley
½ small beet
½ cup pineapple
2 medium green apples
1 sprig fresh mint
½ medium lemon, peeled
Juice.

Red apples can also be used;
these will add extra sweetness.

I fancy myself as a foodie, because man, oh man, do I love to eat. I come from a Southern family, so my taste leans more toward butter and sugar than veggies; if they're battered in cornmeal and fried, then I'm in! Growing up, I was interested in creative preparations of vegetables that were able to mask their flavor. Then a few years ago, I had a juice that changed it all for me—a mix that's better than any po' boy you'll ever eat. The vegetables in their purest form are refreshing and palate cleansing, while the sweet notes of the fruits and mint make it both quenching and intoxicating. Now I can get my dose of veggies in a delicious way and feel proud doing it. And boy, does is counter the guilt I feel when pulling out the ice cream.

—Blake Lively, actor

JUICE BOOST: FAT IS YOUR FRIEND

A dash of healthy, unprocessed fat added to a juice can help with the absorption of nutrients from vegetables and fruits, making your drink truly liquid gold. The powerful antioxidant carotenoids found in green foods (like spinach and kale) and red and orange plants (like carrots, bell peppers, watermelon, and grapefruit) are fat soluble, so a dash of seed or nut oil in the drink helps them get into your system. (Or a fatty fruit: Add avocado to a blend of tomatoes, carrots, or bell peppers, and you'll absorb up to five times more of the carotenoids, lycopene, and beta-carotene.)

Fats and oils can also add a host of their own intrinsic nutritional benefits to your supplement-in-a-cup—oils are a great source of energy for your body, trumping sugar in efficiency and impact—and most raw oils come with a host of extra benefits.

Stirring a spoon of seed oil into your juice or quickly blending your fresh juice with avocado or a spoon of coconut oil to give a thicker texture are two easy ways to add some fat to your glass. Fats slow down absorption of nutrients: This is a bonus when it comes to slowing and stabilizing the impact of juice's sugars on your blood, though some may find the effect of untouched juice more uplifting. As always, the final choice is up to you: Listen to your body and see how you feel in the hour or so after your drink.

FLAXSEED OIL is a rich source of omega-3 fatty acids, essential nutrients that we must get from food and that most of us are deficient in. These fatty acids benefit every cell in the body, helping to improve blood circulation and reduce inflammation, and benefitting hair, nails, and skin. Flaxseed oil is often added to juices in nutritional healing programs because the fatty acids help to carry beta-carotene into the bloodstream to increase the body's immune response. It is fairly delicate: Any heat used in processing damages its structure, so purchase cold-pressed oil from your store's refrigerator case. Keep it in your fridge and, once open, use quickly; within eight weeks is recommended so it does not go rancid. **Try: Stirring 1 teaspoon flaxseed oil into your fresh juice.**

JUICY TIP

Coconut oil is quite shelf stable and can be stored in a cupboard. In cool temperatures, coconut oil turns from a liquid to a solid. You can gently heat the oil on a stovetop (a couple of minutes on very low heat) back to liquid form before adding to a cold—or room temperature—beverage to avoid lumps.

COCONUT OIL is an extremely healing food with antiviral, antifungal, and antimicrobial properties that actually promote weight loss and help to regulate thyroid function and normalize blood sugar. It contains medium-chain fatty acids (MCFAs), which, unlike the long-chain fatty acids found in other veggie oils, don't accumulate as fat in the body. MCFAs are sent directly to the liver to be converted to energy. This energy boost helps improve sluggish metabolisms and manage weight gain. Lauric acid, a substance also found in human breast milk, makes up most of the MCFAs found in coconut oil. It converts to monolaurin in the body, which has been linked to increased immunity. This multitasking master is also a supreme all-over moisturizer, massage oil, makeup remover, and hair hydrator. **Try: Blending 1 teaspoon to 1 tablespoon raw, cold-processed coconut oil into your juice. Blend for under 30 seconds to preserve optimal nutrients in the juice.**

AVOCADO'S unsaturated fat contains oleic acid, which research shows activates the brain area that increases the feeling of satiety. **Try: Blending a scoop of avocado into a green or vegetable-based juice to give it satisfying, smoothie texture.**

All these things can of course be easily added into smoothies, too, plus one more fat-rich addition:

NUT BUTTER. A spoonful of almond butter, peanut butter, cashew butter, as well as seed butters like hemp butter and tahini (sesame seed butter), adds a fabulous range of flavors and fueling fats to a blended drink. Look for minimally processed butters with no added sugar—and seek out a raw variety if possible, to avoid the damaging effects of the highly heated oils. Feeling ambitious? With a masticating juicer, a high-speed blender, or even a food processor, plus a little patience, you can even make your own butter from nothing but raw nuts.

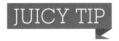

JUICY TIP

Fats don't have to be added to the drink itself; many people swear by a handful of raw nuts alongside their juice to maximize the nutritional uptake.

I have been the pickiest eater my entire life. Sadly I hated vegetables growing up. Since cutting meat and dairy entirely from my diet years ago, I was faced with a big dilemma of what to eat in addition to my much loved diet of rice, beans, and avocados. Once I discovered juicing, my whole world changed. I absolutely love vegetable juices and have incorporated them into my daily diet, and I feel fantastic as a result.

—**Famke Janssen, actor**

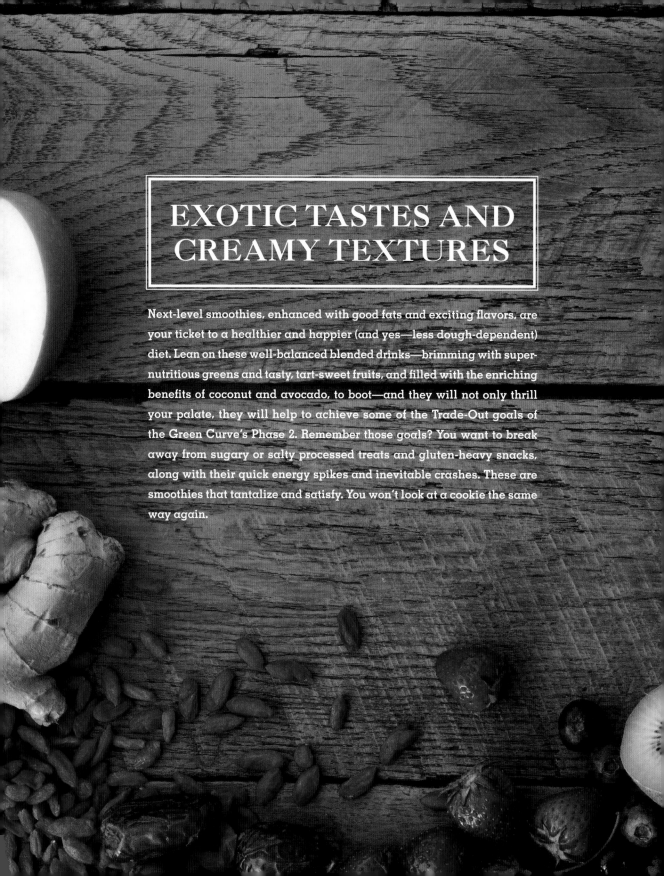

EXOTIC TASTES AND CREAMY TEXTURES

Next-level smoothies, enhanced with good fats and exciting flavors, are your ticket to a healthier and happier (and yes—less dough-dependent) diet. Lean on these well-balanced blended drinks—brimming with super-nutritious greens and tasty, tart-sweet fruits, and filled with the enriching benefits of coconut and avocado, to boot—and they will not only thrill your palate, they will help to achieve some of the Trade-Out goals of the Green Curve's Phase 2. Remember those goals? You want to break away from sugary or salty processed treats and gluten-heavy snacks, along with their quick energy spikes and inevitable crashes. These are smoothies that tantalize and satisfy. You won't look at a cookie the same way again.

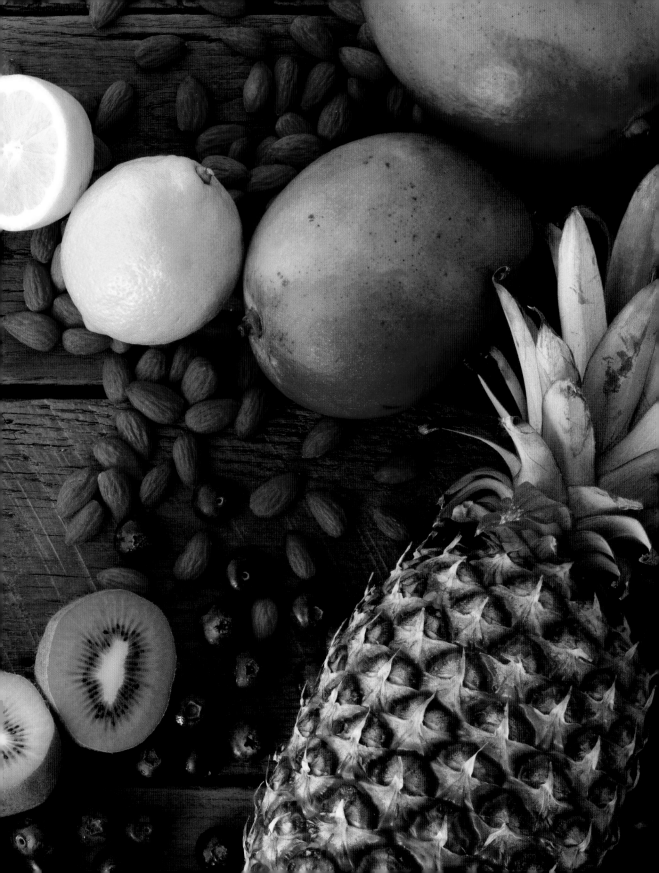

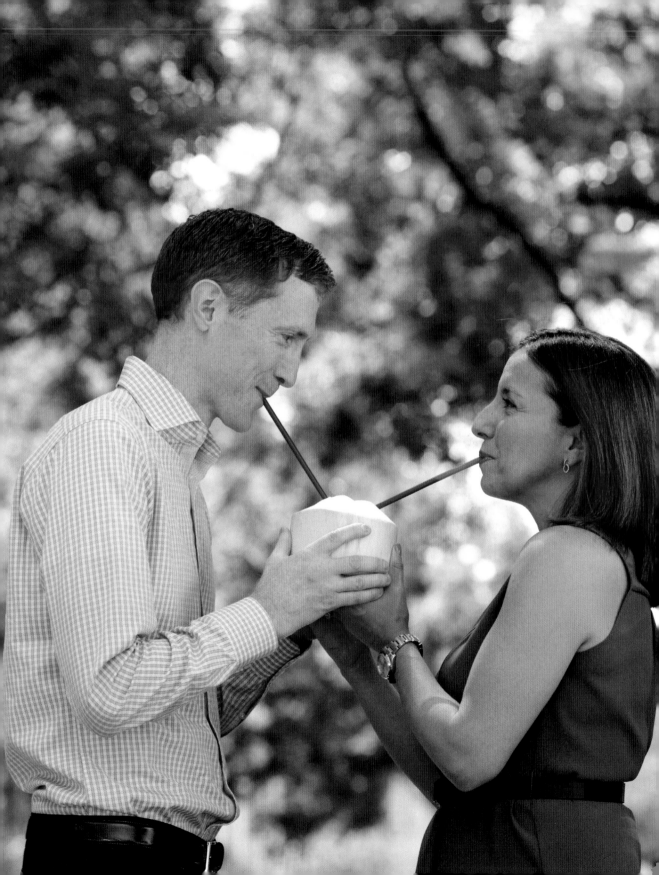

COCO LOVE!

A coconut is one tough nut that we love to crack. Call it guilt-free dessert in a glass, or instant escape to a more tropical state of being. The fragrant, island-evoking flavor of the raw water straight from a fresh, young coconut has a kind of euphoric effect that packaged coconut water, for all its convenience, can never quite achieve. Young coconuts are the white, husk-free variety and have a thin layer of soft, white flesh inside and a reservoir of coconut water.

Raw coconut water is rich in electrolytes, the electrically charged ions that help our cells communicate and that get depleted by hard exercise. It's also high in enzymes that help to detoxify and repair the body, as well as beneficial lauric acid.

Use the refreshing, energizing elixir from young coconuts to make blended drinks and discover how coconuts turn everyday ingredients into a sumptuous treat. Or keep it super simple and eco-aware by sipping the young coconut water straight from the shell: nature's to-go cup.

— CRACK THAT NUT —

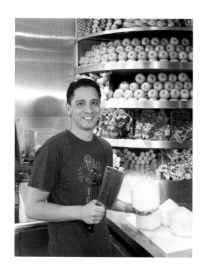

THE TOOLS

A large, sharp knife with a heel

A young coconut (This method works best with young or "green" coconuts.)

THE STEPS

1. Lay coconut on its side, keeping any plastic wrapping on the fruit. (Young coconuts that have had their outer green shell removed are often treated with chemicals to keep their inner shell looking white and pretty. Keeping the plastic wrapper in place as long as possible prevents the toxins from seeping into your cutting surface. These chemicals do not harm the inside of the coconut.)

2. Cut away at pointed top of the coconut until the round inner cap is revealed. This will be the "lid" of the coconut.

3. Hit the edge of this lid with your knife at a 45-degree angle so that it pops up.

4. Use the heel of the knife to wedge the lid up.

5. Pour out the water. (If the water has a pink tinge, it has gone bad. Discard the coconut and its water!)

6. Use a flexible spatula to dig out the soft coconut meat, which can then be eaten on its own or blended into smoothies. A coconut scraper or "de-meater" tool makes scooping even easier.

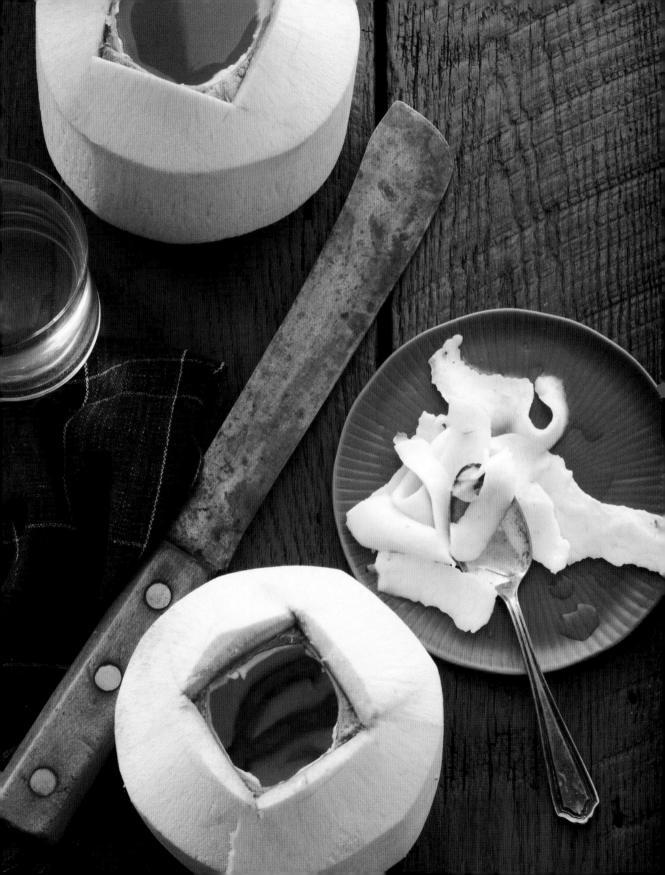

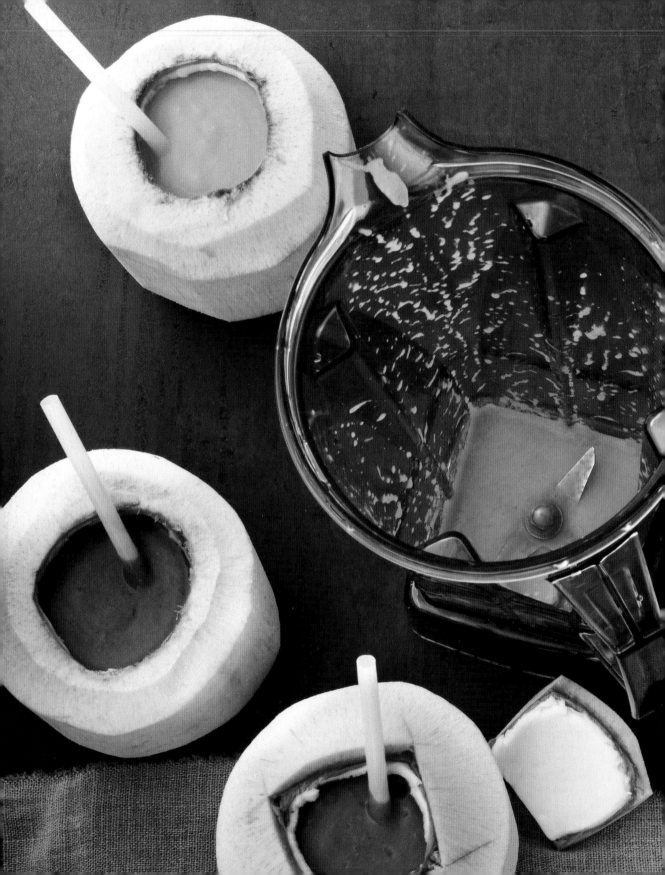

Coconut puts a rich spin on almost any blended drink. Have fun experimenting with this versatile ingredient to make a satisfying and uplifting breakfast smoothie or anytime snack. Here are our favorite four coco-blend drinks

Kale Kolada

Leafy greens take on a tropical twist when paired with coconut. Add a dash of cinnamon for a sweeter twist.

1 freshly cracked young Thai coconut, water and meat
1 cup spinach
1 cup kale
½ medium banana
Blend.

Carrot Creamsicle

Easy as one-two-three, a touch of sweet carrot brings a surprising and colorful touch to a fresh coco cup.

1 freshly cracked young Thai coconut, water and meat
1 medium carrot
Blend.

Amazon Acaí

The antioxidant power of the Amazonian berry acaí paired with the decadent creaminess of coconut and banana makes this blend healthy and heavenly.

1 freshly cracked young Thai coconut, water and meat
1 pack frozen acaí
½ medium banana
Blend.
See page 168 for more on acaí and how to use it.

Pacific Pineapple

Pineapple and coconut, the classic beachcomber duo, are enhanced with strawberries' fiber, potassium, and vitamin C.

1 freshly cracked young Thai coconut, water and meat
¼ cup pineapple
¼ cup strawberries
Blend.

JUICY TIP

When selecting young coconuts, be sure to get the most recent ones to arrive at the store and make sure there is no mold or moisture under the plastic wrap.

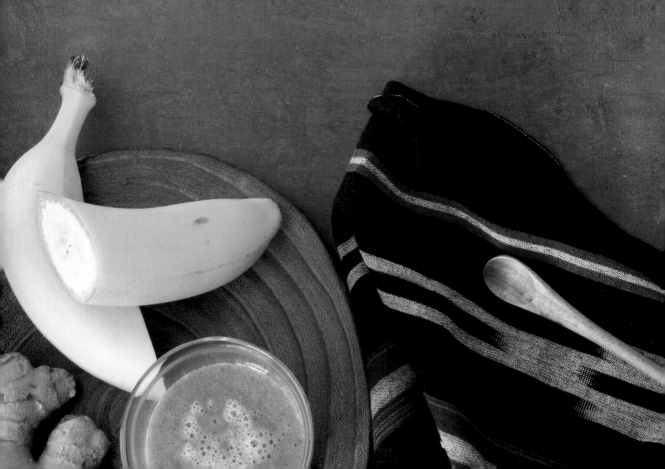

I have a big garden and throw in whatever is in season. I love kale, carrot, spinach, apple, and I even get creative throwing in flax oil, aloe juice, and lemons from the tree in my yard. Having fresh juices is mandatory for me—it is a part of my regular diet.

—Kristen Bell, actor

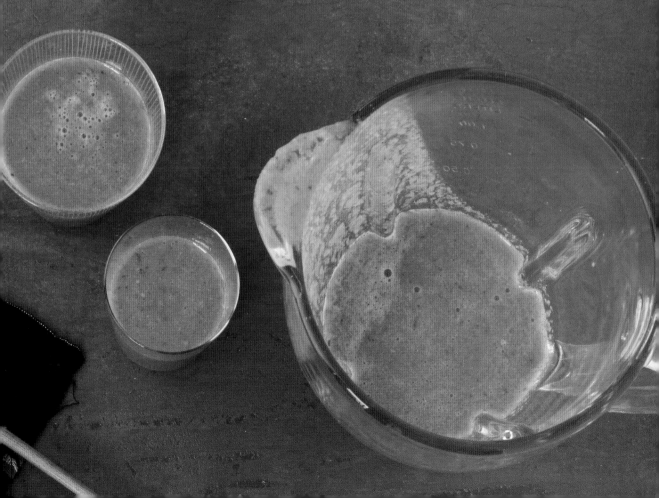

Sweet 'n' Creamy Greens

¼ medium avocado
1 cup kale
1 cup almond milk
½ medium banana
3 medium dates, pitted
½ cup ice
Blend.

CocoBliss

1 freshly cracked young Thai coconut, water and meat
¼ medium avocado
Blend.

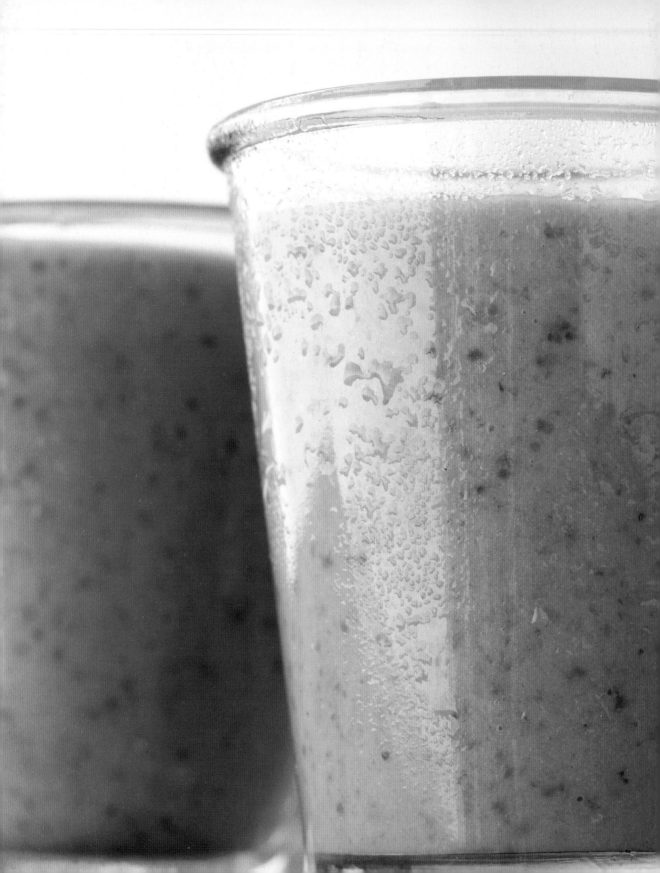

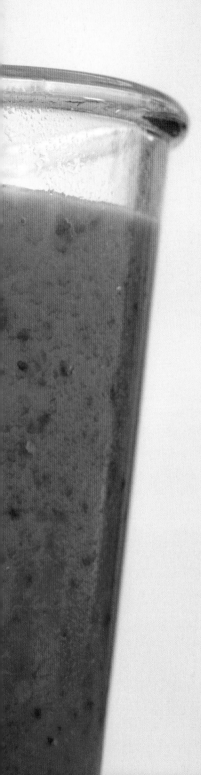

Berry Cherry

Tart flavors have a sneaky way of perking up your palate. The acerola cherry, also called the Amazon cherry, has ten times the vitamin C of orange juice—great for immunity—and a refreshing, tart citrus flavor. Here, it mingles with raspberries, which are loaded with antioxidants.

½ cup acerola cherries
½ cup raspberries
½ medium frozen banana
1 cup fresh orange juice
Blend.

Mango Tango

Like its dark leafy green cousin, kale, Swiss chard is a nutritional winner delivering a jolt of supercharged vitamins and minerals. If you prefer less intense green flavor, stick with the smaller leaves, which are sweeter.

2 leaves Swiss chard
1 cup mango
½ medium lime, peeled
1 cup filtered water
½ cup ice
Blend.

JUICY TIP

Acerola can be found as a frozen fruit and also as a freeze-dried powder that can be added to all kinds of smoothies for a nutritious enhancement. If acerola is out of reach, use ordinary fresh or frozen cherries; they will have a sweeter taste so adjust the recipe if you like by diluting the orange juice with water.

Luscious Cup

Sometimes the most unlikely ingredients make the tastiest smoothies or juices. A happy accident led us to this strangely tasty combination of creamy, spicy, tropical, and tart.

1 cup mango
1 cup spinach
½ medium orange, peeled
½ medium banana
1 cup soy milk
1 inch fresh gingerroot, peeled
Blend.

Fruity Fiesta

Ginger gives this green smoothie a spicy kick. Keep the potent root on hand to quickly boost the flavor of any juice or blended drink. Hint: Ginger lasts longer if you store it in your crisper drawer in a zip-top bag or vegetable storage bag. If you need to sweeten your smoothie, try adding a date or two.

1 cup spinach
½ cup parsley
½ medium orange, peeled
½ medium apple
1 inch fresh gingerroot, peeled
½ medium frozen banana
½ medium lemon, peeled
1 cup filtered water
Blend.

Todo Bueno

This seductive drink contains seven of our favorite things. It gets its beautiful flecks of red by spiking a medley of everyday fruits and vegetables with a sneak preview of a Phase 3 superfood—the tiny goji berry, known to some as wolfberry.

1 cup spinach
2 tablespoons soaked goji berries
½ cup strawberries
½ medium banana
½ medium avocado
1 cup hemp milk
3 dates, pitted
Blend.

See page 204 for more on goji berries.

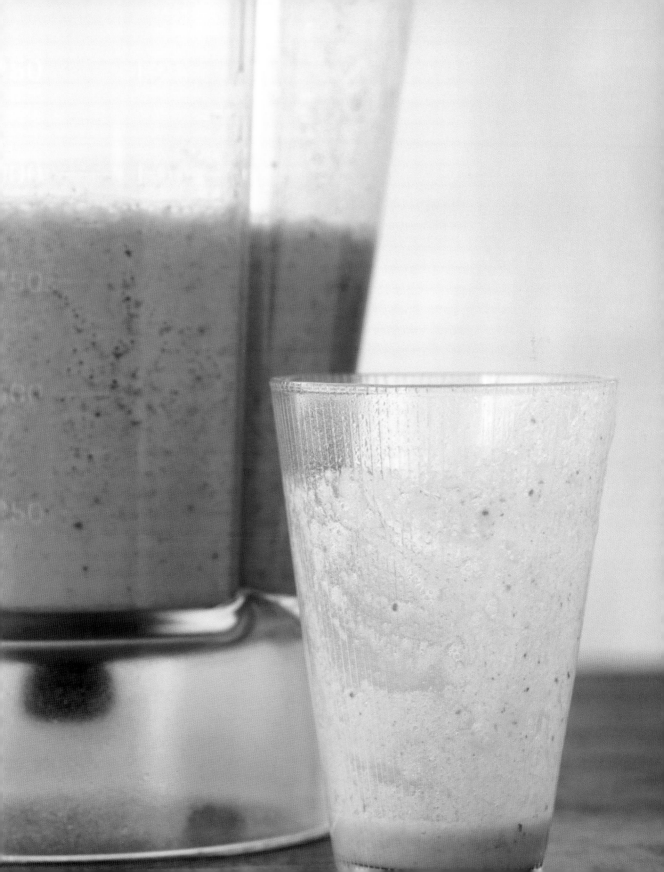

HEMP SEEDS

THE NATURAL WONDER OF HEMP

Sometimes you want something extra in your cup—a boost of protein after a workout or a balanced dose of protein and fat to make it from breakfast to lunch without crashing. Once, the only easy-to-find option for powering up a smoothie was a massive tub of bodybuilder protein powder. Today, things have changed, as next-gen smoothie makers go back to basics and seek out earthier alternatives: raw, whole-food sources of protein that have not been processed by heat or enhanced with chemical sweeteners or additives.

Our favorite all-natural way to add protein and fat to a smoothie is hemp seed. This mild and nutty-tasting ingredient has one of the most well-rounded nutritional profiles of any plant food and is one of nature's richest sources of plant protein. It's low allergenic—unlike many whey and soy proteins—easily digestible, and blends well into drinks with an appealing taste. (And unlike sweetened powders, it works well in green-based and savory blended drinks.)

Hemp Protein Buzz

A satisfying smoothie that will keep you fueled, this can be made extra good with homemade hemp milk, as described in Phase 3 (page 199).

1 cup hemp milk
1 scoop protein powder
¼ cup blueberries
¼ cup strawberries
½ medium frozen banana
3 medium dates, pitted
½ cup ice
Blend.

Hemp seeds come in many forms, including the raw, hulled seeds, concentrated protein powder, luscious seed butter, cold-pressed oil, and creamy hemp milk, giving you endless options to play with. Not to mention, the complete hemp plant is a natural wonder, providing us with ecofriendly textiles and paper, plastic alternatives and building materials, herbal medicines—and more.

Start with a bag of hulled seeds (also sometimes called hemp hearts) and add 2 tablespoons to your smoothie. Grind them in the blender alone before adding any other ingredients to make the nutrients most absorbable. (A clean coffee grinder can help if your blender fails at the job.) If you like the taste, and need more protein, try a raw hemp protein powder, which is made by concentrating the protein from hemp, giving you 15 grams or more per serving. The more finely ground the powder, the more you'll probably enjoy it.

And, if you love this simple, whole-food addition to your smoothie, you might also try one of the more complex, "sprouted" plant-protein powders on the market that mix raw and unprocessed protein from an array of seeds, peas, and gluten-free grains, often in delicious combinations.

HEMP POWER

Raw hemp seeds are about 35 percent protein, with a complete array of amino acids that are easily digested by the body, and about 45 percent fat, with a perfect ratio of omega-3 to omega-6 essential fatty acids, along with the rare "super" polyunsaturated fats, gamma-linolenic acid (GLA) and stearidonic acid (SDA), and the "beautifying" oil of omega 9-fatty acids. Lots of enzymes, low antinutrients, and about 20 trace minerals make it a true super seed.

THE SCOOP ON PROTEIN POWDERS

Navigating the complex world of protein powders is challenging. What's healthy and what's potentially harmful? These foods fall under the category of "supplements" and their claims and ingredients aren't regulated by the FDA. Some muscle-building powders have been found to contain high levels of heavy metals. Look for the most natural and least-processed product you can. Whey, from dairy, is best if cold-processed and from cows free of rBGH (growth hormone) or better yet, fully organic, with no added sugar. If using a powder containing soy protein isolate, just as with soy milk it is wise to seek one that is non-GMO.

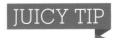

Store your hemp seeds or powder in the fridge to ensure the fats do not turn rancid; use within three months.

Coconut oil helps you absorb the omega-3 fatty acids in hemp twice as effectively. Try a smoothie featuring both those ingredients.

I make protein shakes after I work out—it's a really easy way of getting all my protein in as well as chucking in all the other stuff I need. I love eating spinach, but my wife, Thara, manages to find a sneaky way of putting it into my shakes so I don't even know how many extra nutrients I'm getting. And I love berries—I put a lot of them into my shakes.

—Jay Sean, singer-songwriter

ACAÍ

Purple Power: Who doesn't like to consume the color purple? It's not only great for you—dark red, blue, and violet fruits are some of nature's wonder stuffs—it is also, frankly, fun. Acaí grows wild on the banks of the Amazon and has long been a staple food in Brazil, where it's eaten in puree form as part of a savory meal, and where surfers throw the frozen slush into fruit smoothies as a after-surf refueling.

An exotic relative of our blueberry and cranberry, acaí berries are over-flowing with antioxidants (of the anthocyanin variety, just like red wine) and healthy fats with not a drop of sugar in sight. When Juice Genera-tion first introduced acaí in 2000, Brazilian expats were the primary takers, scooping up our chilled acaí breakfast bowls: One step beyond a smoothie, an acaí bowl features frozen acaí pulp, granola, banana, and other fruits and veggies. Soon, the pre- and postworkout crowds caught wind and started using acaí bowls to charge up before—or recover from—Spinning and yoga. Today, we sell hundreds of acaí bowls every day to athletes, executives, and anyone looking for a refreshing fuel-up of raw ingredi-ents that won't leave them feeling bogged down and groggy. Replete with protein and good fat, vitamins and antioxidants, these bowls will kick-start the day or carry you from midafternoon to dinner. Skip the bagel and go for the bowl.

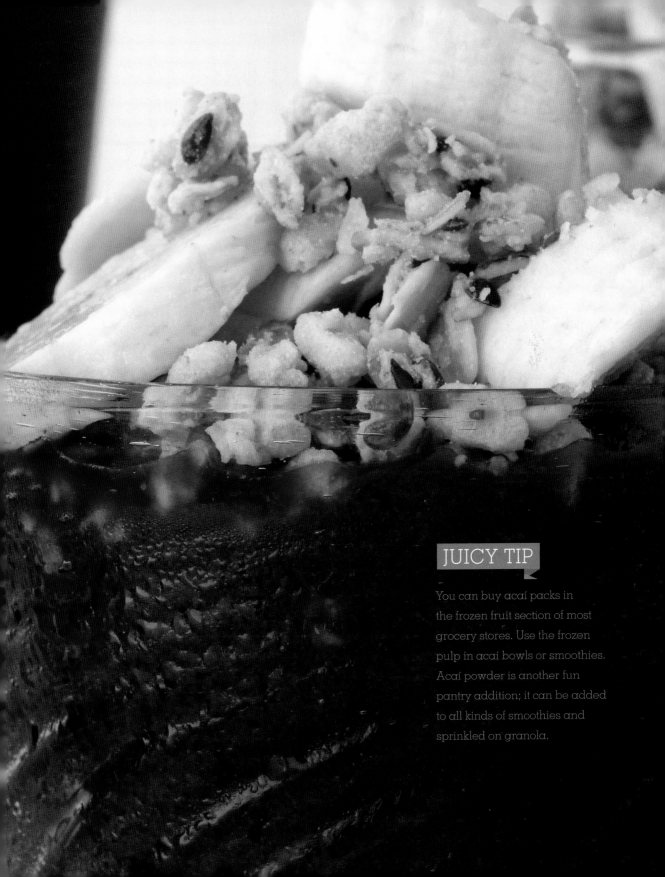

JUICY TIP

You can buy acaí packs in
the frozen fruit section of most
grocery stores. Use the frozen
pulp in acaí bowls or smoothies.
Acaí powder is another fun
pantry addition; it can be added
to all kinds of smoothies and
sprinkled on granola.

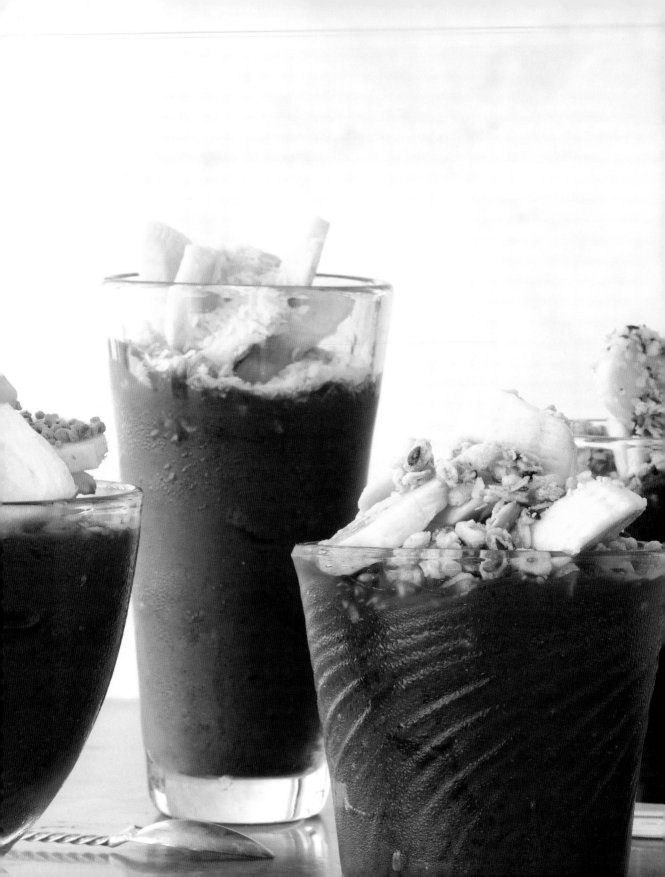

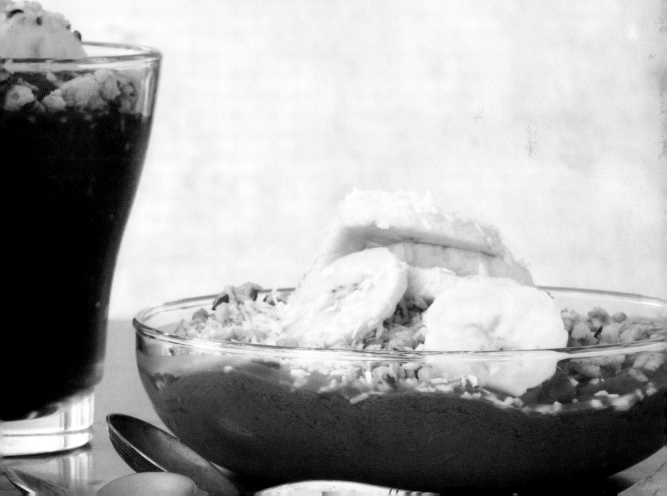

Our typical day at the Alvin Ailey American Dance Theater is extremely intense. We start with a class in the morning, and from twelve until seven we're in rehearsal. We are basically physical for a full workday, so it's really important that we power our bodies with great food. Almost all the Ailey dancers juice, and I usually have an Amazing Green Acaí Bowl in the morning. It's a great way to get a full breakfast in a really healthy way, and it's quick and easy. If I guarantee that I get my greens in the morning, I feel like the rest of the day is going to go really well.

—Alicia Graf Mack, dancer, Alvin Ailey American Dance Theater

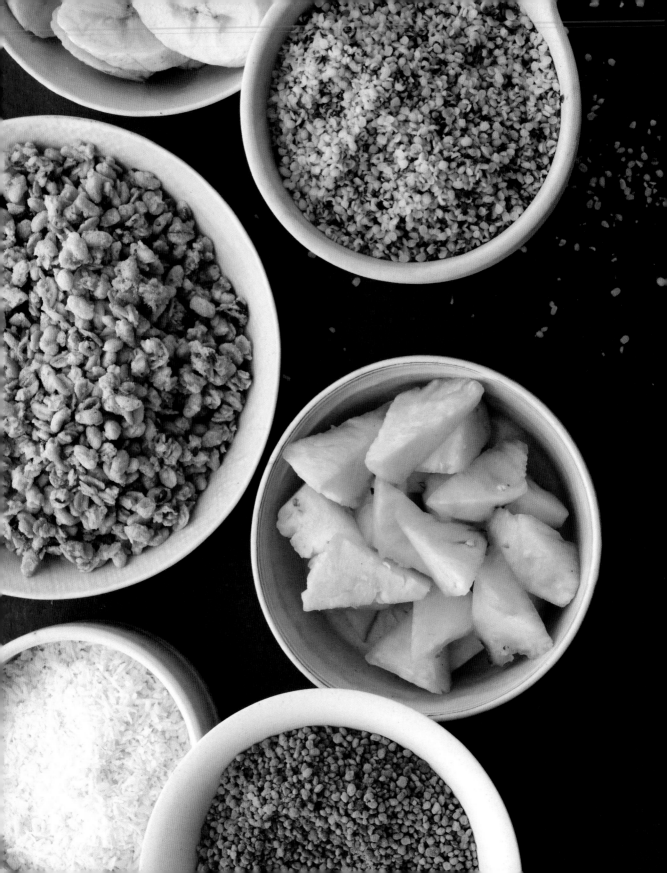

Amazing Green Acaí Bowl

2 packs frozen acaí
½ cup spinach
½ cup kale
½ medium banana
¾ cup almond milk
Blend.

Top with 2 teaspoons hemp seeds, ⅓ medium banana, ¼ cup hemp granola.

Aloha Acaí Bowl

Bee pollen—a food you'll meet properly in Phase 3—adds a hit of ultrawellness to this island-inspired bowl.

2 packs frozen acaí
½ medium banana
¾ cup almond milk
Blend.

Top with 2 teaspoons bee pollen, ½ cup pineapple, ⅓ medium banana, ¼ cup hemp granola.

Hemp Acaí Bowl

Quadruple the hemp and quadruple the goodness. This one will have you dancing, Spinning, and upward-dogging like a pro.

2 packs frozen acaí
1 tablespoon hemp protein
½ medium banana
¾ cup hemp milk
Blend.

Top with ¼ cup hemp granola, ⅓ medium banana, 2 teaspoons hemp seeds.

PB Acaí Bowl

The crunch of cacao nibs on a peanut-buttery blend makes this absolutely joy inducing.

2 packs frozen acaí
1 tablespoon peanut butter
½ medium banana
¾ cup almond milk
Blend.

Top with 2 teaspoons peanut butter, 2 teaspoons cacao nibs, ⅓ medium banana, ¼ cup hemp granola.

Coco Acaí Bowl

Rich and creamy coconut milk makes any blended treat heavenly. Made fresh at home, it is sumptuous. If using canned coconut milk, look for the variety with no additives and better yet, a can with minimal BPAs in its lining.

2 packs frozen acaí
½ medium banana
¾ cup coconut milk
Blend.

Top with dried shredded coconut, ⅓ medium banana, ¼ cup hemp granola.

JUICY TIP

Hemp granola is available at natural food stores and features hemp seeds mixed into a crunchy, oat, and seed base. It's easy to make your own, and you can use gluten-free oats if you choose.

phase

ULTRA GREEN: THE FULL FEEL-GOOD EFFECT

This final phase takes you on a journey into the next frontier of juicing and blending, where nature's abundant gifts are used to maximum effect. Juices in this phase feature super-green ingredients that have powerful nourishing and detoxifying qualities. You'll discover how good it feels (and tastes) to make fresh nut milks from scratch; you'll become your own healer, making DIY tonics for the days you feel under the weather and instant wellness shots to keep you boosted year-round. Then, you'll become a master of smoothies using homemade milks, and get adventurous by enhancing these whole-food drinks with superfood ingredients for intriguing flavors and extraprotective benefits. There will be times of coure when you're drawn to making a luscious drink that stands on its own without greens (like an almond-cacao smoothie or a spice-touched nut milk). These drinks also have lots of important nutrients and are fabulous with or without greens.

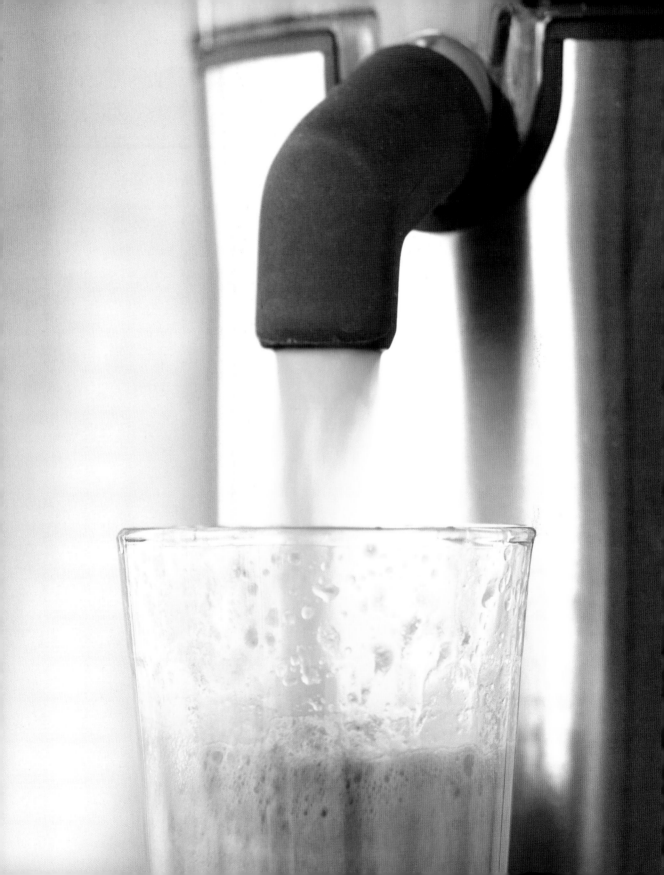

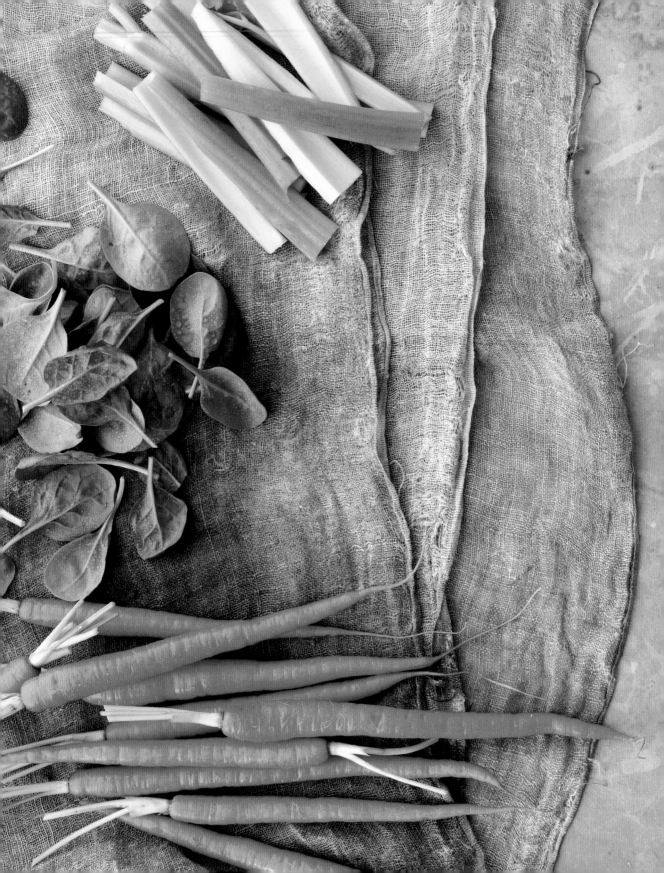

Just try to make a baseline habit of one green-filled drink a day—with some room for treats here and there.

THE TRADE-OUT: In Phase 1 you replaced a caffeinated beverage with a juice or smoothie; Phase 2 was all about ditching a sugary or gluten-heavy snack for a produce-packed drink; now it's about using juices and smoothies strategically, as a tool to see you through each day. Juicing and blending can fit into your unique lifestyle. Perhaps you'll turn to a liquid breakfast—or dinner—if you're feeling puffy and heavy from recent indulgences and want to start or end the day lighter (and sleep better, too). Or maybe you're strapped for time to prepare a healthy meal and want to drink your veggies on the go. This is not about liquefying your diet completely—remember, juicing and blending is about adding, not subtracting. Instead, strategically use juices and smoothies to add balance to your life. Rushing to the airport for an early flight? Drop five supercharged ingredients in the blender and pour the results into a to-go cup; this will serve you better and take you farther (no carb crash later) than a latte and muffin before takeoff. Pushing through a heavy business dinner with nary a lettuce leaf in sight? Find equilibrium again with a green juice for breakfast. Gearing up for a big evening party? Drink a juice or smoothie for lunch to give your digestive system a break before diving into the festivities.

Bonus: Adding detoxifying ingredients will help you cleanse your system more efficiently on a daily basis.

Juice Smarts: When in doubt, go green. A good ratio to aim for most days is 3 parts veggie to 1 part fruit.

PHASE 3
BUYING GUIDE

Your Green Curve goal in Phase 3 is to make a green-filled drink every day. We'll call this a 90 percent green drink habit—to keep it realistic with a little wiggle room. Whether it's a juice, a smoothie, or a superfood smoothie that you enhance with a handful of greens or perhaps a green superfood powder, and whether you pick your recipes entirely from the ones listed here, or reuse favorites from Phases 1 and 2, we simply want you to get your greens in every day!

VEGETABLES

- COLLARD GREENS
- CILANTRO
- BOK CHOY
- DANDELION GREENS
- JALEPENO PEPPER
- FRESH WHEATGRASS
- BURDOCK ROOT
- TURMERIC ROOT

FRUIT

- POMEGRANATE
- PAPAYA
- FROZEN ARONIA BERRIES
- PITAYA
- MANGOSTEEN

PANTRY

- RAW NUTS
- GREEN TEA
- PINK HIMALAYAN SALT
- RAW CACAO POWDER
- SEA BUCKTHORN
- BLUE-GREEN ALGAE
- MACA ROOT POWDER
- CAYENNE PEPPER
- TURMERIC POWDER
- CARDAMOM
- VANILLA BEAN
- BEE POLLEN
- SPIRULINA
- CHIA SEEDS
- IRISH MOSS

RX

- LIQUID ECHINACEA
- VITAMIN C

PHASE 3 JUICES: ULTRA GREEN AND DETOXIFYING

Now that any initial resistance to greens-in-a-glass has faded, infuse your juice with some major green players: plants and roots that are a little less commonly used—and that are more intense in flavor than cucumbers or carrots. We've made it easy to drink your dandelion, watercress, wheatgrass, collards, and burdock—something you can feel very good about, because your liver and blood cells will thank you! Then, open the spice cabinet and doctor your juices with turmeric, cayenne, and salt—hits of enhanced flavor with surprising, curative properties.

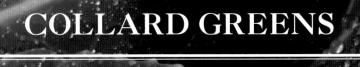

COLLARD GREENS

Introducing juicing's up-and-coming superfood: The humble, dark green collard leaf is not especially enticing, but it wins our award for Next Big Thing because it grows abundantly close to home and delivers a ridiculously high quota of nutrition per calorie, including tons of vitamin C and some remarkable anticancer properties. We predict this Southern-food staple will play a leading role in the burgeoning juice revolution, as people fall in love with its affordable price, its ease-of-cultivation for the home gardener, and the large volume of juice it produces. (Not to mention its efficacy in restoring health: Collards have been associated with reduction of inflammation-related diseases like Crohn's disease, irritable bowl syndrome, and rheumatoid arthritis.) On its own, collard juice has a strong flavor, so mix it with the right companions to temper its potency and enjoy its benefits. And as with all deep-green leaves, rotate them over the course of a month rather than relying on them every single day.

Collard Cooler

Mixed with cucumber, citrus, and apple, as well as the neutral flavors of cucumber and celery, the green goodness goes down easy. Adjust amounts of lemon and lime to taste.

2 leaves collard greens
2½ medium green apples
½ medium cucumber
2 stalks celery
½ medium lemon, peeled
½ medium lime, peeled
Juice.

Zesty Green

Collard greens have a similar nutritional profile to that juicing superstar, kale, but they produce significantly more juice, making them not only supremely healthy, but also supremely economical. This mix, enhanced by the detoxifying boost of cilantro, has a delicious sweet-spicy kick.

2 leaves collard greens
¼ cup cilantro
1½ medium green apples
3 medium carrots
¼ medium cucumber
1 inch fresh gingerroot, peeled
Juice.

Mega Green

Consider this concoction the granddaddy of green—leaves galore with only a kiss of fruit in the form of tart green apple and lemon. For die-hard juicers dedicated to keeping sugars low, this drink is a failsafe staple.

2 leaves collard greens
1 cup spinach
2 leaves romaine
¼ medium cucumber
3 stalks celery
2 medium green apples
½ medium lemon, peeled
Juice.

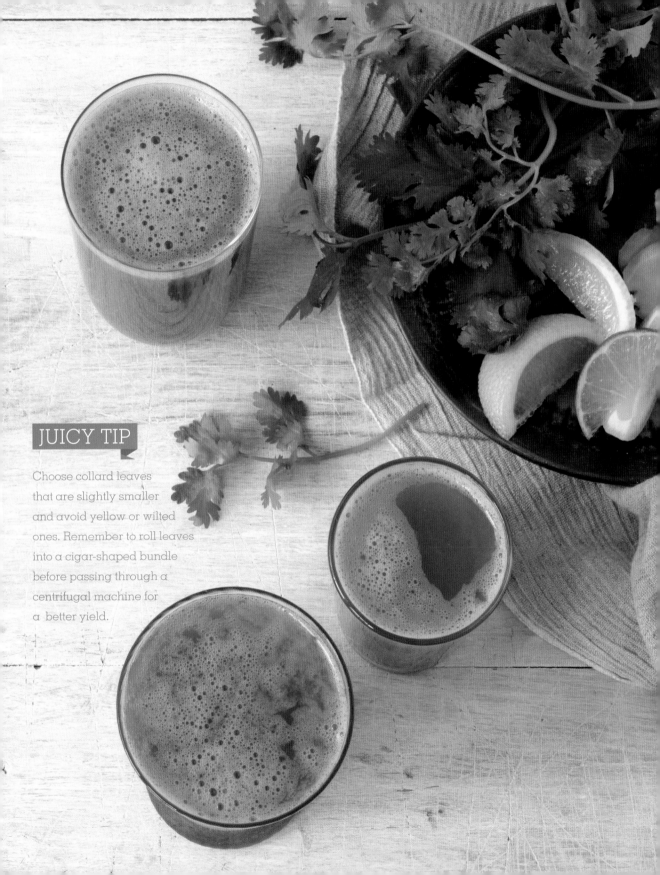

JUICY TIP

Choose collard leaves
that are slightly smaller
and avoid yellow or wilted
ones. Remember to roll leaves
into a cigar-shaped bundle
before passing through a
centrifugal machine for
a better yield.

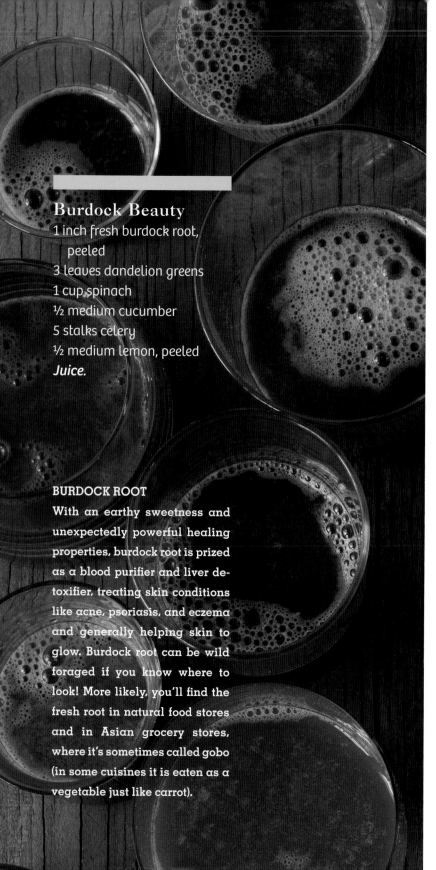

Burdock Beauty

1 inch fresh burdock root, peeled
3 leaves dandelion greens
1 cup spinach
½ medium cucumber
5 stalks celery
½ medium lemon, peeled
Juice.

BURDOCK ROOT

With an earthy sweetness and unexpectedly powerful healing properties, burdock root is prized as a blood purifier and liver detoxifier, treating skin conditions like acne, psoriasis, and eczema and generally helping skin to glow. Burdock root can be wild foraged if you know where to look! More likely, you'll find the fresh root in natural food stores and in Asian grocery stores, where it's sometimes called gobo (in some cuisines it is eaten as a vegetable just like carrot).

The Detoxifier

2 leaves dandelion greens
¼ cup watercress
1 cup kale
1 cup spinach
½ cup parsley
½ medium pear
½ medium cucumber
4 stalks celery
1 inch fresh gingerroot, peeled
½ medium lemon, peeled
Juice.

DANDELION GREENS

Bitter greens are what juice is made for—the stuff that's hard to eat, but easier to drink. Dandelion leaf deserves the effort. The prolific weed—it's found in the wilds everywhere, but is particularly bountiful in the spring, when the body is due for an after-winter tune-up—boosts the gallbladder's production of bile, which tones the liver. It's fine to pick dandelion greens that are growing wild—if you are sure they are not near lawns or other areas treated with pesticides, or on the shoulders of roads exposed to exhaust fumes.

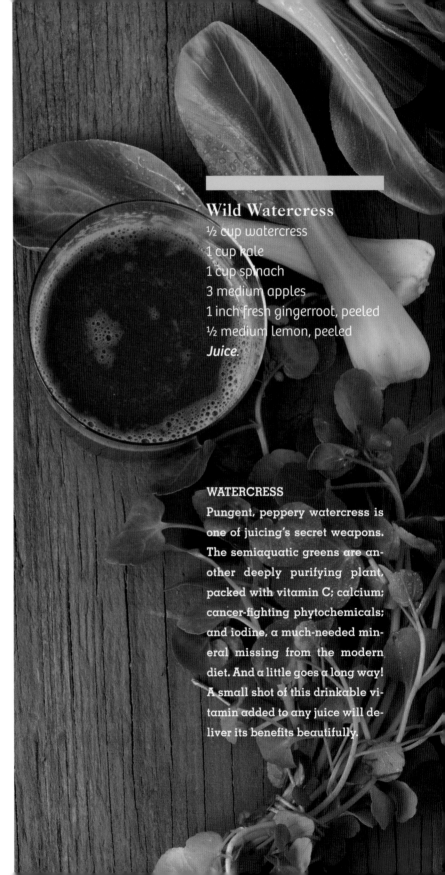

Jade Joy

2 stalks bok choy
1 cup spinach
1 cup parsley
1 medium green apple
3 stalks celery
¼ medium lemon, peeled
Juice.

Wild Watercress

½ cup watercress
1 cup kale
1 cup spinach
3 medium apples
1 inch fresh gingerroot, peeled
½ medium lemon, peeled
Juice.

BOK CHOY

Bok choy is a leafy Chinese cabbage similar to collards in its makeup and boasting all the benefits of cruciferous vegetables, but with a paler color and significantly milder taste. The veggie's gentle flavor, nutritional makeup, and juicing output—each head produces lots of liquid—makes it an ideal base for many juice combinations. When you include bok choy in your juicing recipes, you're infusing your body with anticancer compounds, beta-carotene, folate, plus your daily requirements of vitamins A, C, and K.

WATERCRESS

Pungent, peppery watercress is one of juicing's secret weapons. The semiaquatic greens are another deeply purifying plant, packed with vitamin C; calcium; cancer-fighting phytochemicals; and iodine, a much-needed mineral missing from the modern diet. And a little goes a long way! A small shot of this drinkable vitamin added to any juice will deliver its benefits beautifully.

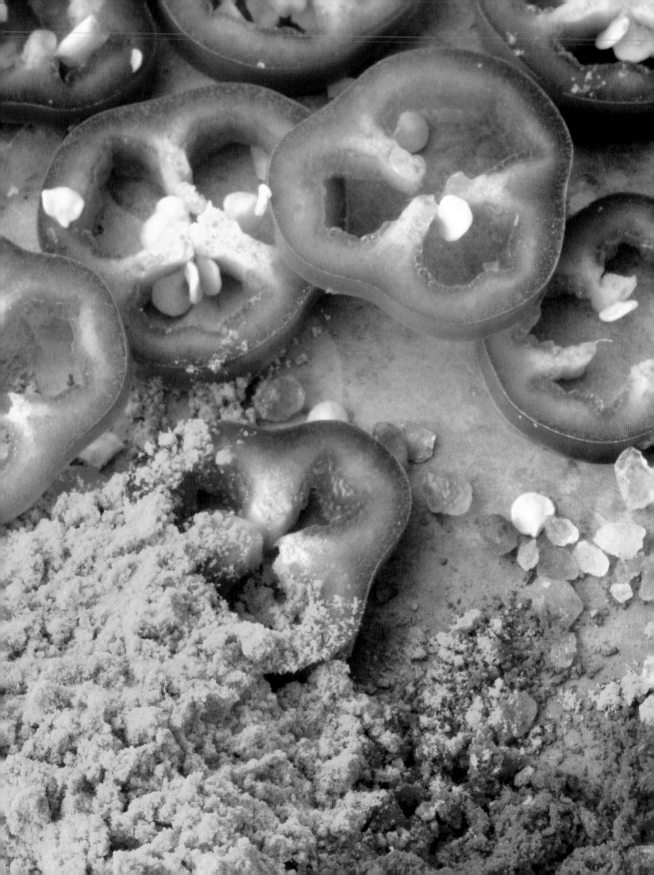

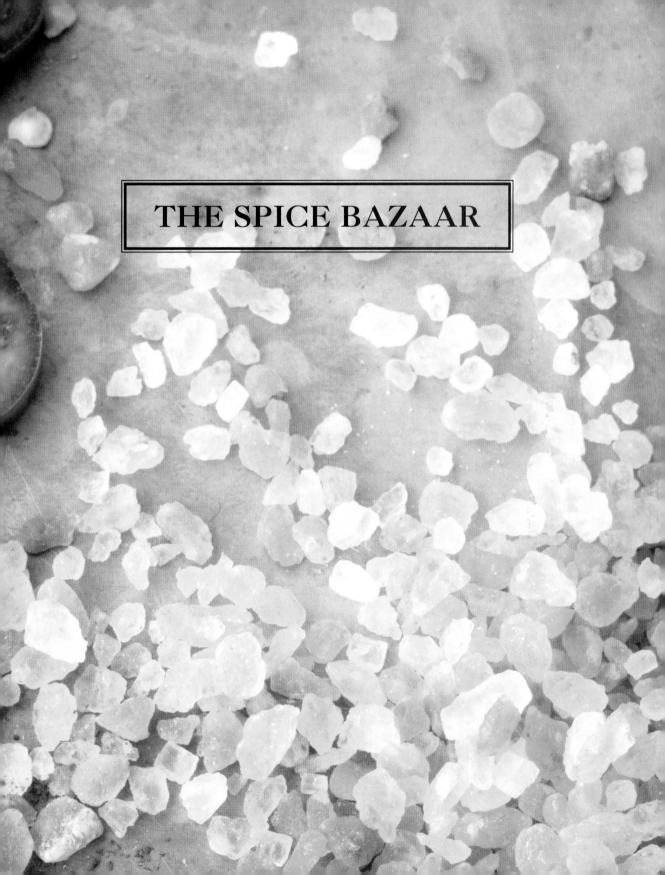

THE SPICE BAZAAR

Cayenne Kick

1 inch fresh gingerroot, peeled
1½ medium apples
5 medium carrots
½ medium lemon, peeled
Juice.

Top with a pinch of cayenne pepper.

Golden Goddess

1 inch fresh turmeric root, peeled
1 cup kale
4 medium carrots
1½ medium apples
3 stalks celery
Juice.

Piña Piquante

½ medium jalapeño
1 cup pineapple
2 medium oranges, peeled
¼ cup cilantro
Juice.

Give your juice a new twist in one simple step by exploring the spice bazaar inside your kitchen cabinets and stealing savory ingredients from your favorite cuisines. With a (moderate) dose of spices and salts, you can add surprising boosts of flavor and health-promoting kicks to your drinks.

CAYENNE PEPPER

The slightest pinch of this hotter-than-hot, orange-red pepper will add a touch of fire to your daily juice. Though its heat may tell you otherwise, cayenne contains a plant compound called capsaicin that has anti-inflammatory properties, which helps achy joints and muscles feel better. The warming effects of cayenne are often used in immunity-boosting elixirs to ward off colds—and it's also proven to be good for your heart. Start small—one tiny shake will do it—and dial up the cayenne if you dare!

TURMERIC

The gorgeous, saffron hue of turmeric is a joyful addition in any kind of cooking. The fresh root found at health food stores and Asian markets is even more of a pleasure to use than the powder—slice into the ginger-like root and you'll be dazzled by its vibrant orange interior. Turmeric, which has a slightly earthy, mildly mustardy, and a gingery taste, is considered a "nutritional medicinal"—a food that has high-level health, wellness, and beautifying effects—and has been used for thousands of years in India's cuisine and medicine. Turmeric is now understood in the West to be a powerful anti-inflammatory wonder herb that delivers a full spectrum of benefits, from liver supporting to immune helping and more. A small shake of turmeric powder can be substituted if the root is not available.

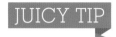

JUICY TIP

Look for firm, ripe jalapeños with shiny skin. If the juice seems too hot, slice the pepper open and scrape out the seeds first. Store unwashed in the fridge, in a paper bag or wrapped in paper towel.

JALAPEÑO

Borrow this essential element from Mexican cooking and in a snap you'll add an energizing shot of heat to a green or fruity juice. Pair it with cilantro for an extra Latin-inspired twist. The freshly extracted capsaicin oil contains important minerals and helps with brain aches like migraines and sinus headaches.

Fresh turmeric root is a humble-looking ingredient that is truly a health and wellness powerhouse. Often sourced from Hawaii, and appearing similar to gingerroot from the outside—although sometimes sold as tiny, individual roots—its gorgeous orange flesh can be juiced and added to smoothies. I consider it a powerful anti-inflammatory ingredient that is a modern-life must-have, and predict it will become as familiar in our kitchens as gingerroot is now. Just be careful in handling it—turmeric is famous as a natural clothing dye for good reason!

—**Amy Myers, MD, functional medicine clinician and educator**

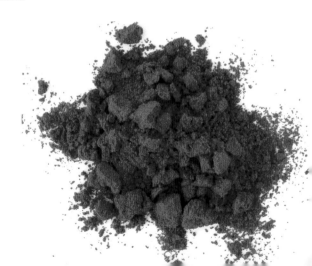

PINK
HIMALAYAN SALT

This pink crystal is a hero product in the raw food world. Sourced from the Himalayan mountains that have formed it over many millions of years, and featuring a precious mix of the 84 trace minerals that our bodies need to function, in extremely absorbable form, Himalayan salt is an ultrapure food source that is sometimes called *white gold*. Small amounts of salt are necessary for our bodies, but it's the unprocessed kind that our cells crave—not the regular table and cooking salt, which is heat-processed (altering its natural structure) and chemically enhanced to prevent caking and drying. Try a hit of Himalayan salt in these vegetable-rich blends to take your juice in a savory new direction and get the full benefit from this unique commodity.

Salsa Samba

Like the most delectable pineapple salsa, this juice is a gustatory joy ride, hitting taste bud hot spots: sweet, salty, and spicy.

2 cups pineapple
½ medium jalapeño
1 cup kale
1 cup spinach
½ cup parsley
3 stalks celery
Juice.

Top with a pinch of pink Himalayan salt.

Hack That Juice! Each salt-enriched juice can be easily hacked into a savory smoothie by adding a quarter of ripe avocado.

The Lift-Off

Here, four players from the leafy green wonder team mingle with the satisfying seasonings of lemon, ginger, and pink Himalayan super salt—like a luscious green soup in a glass.

2 leaves Swiss chard
2 leaves collard greens
1 cup kale
1 cup spinach
½ medium cucumber
1 inch fresh gingerroot, peeled
½ medium lemon, peeled
Juice.

Top with a pinch of pink Himalayan salt.

Carrot Spice

A twist on a classic combo, carrot and ginger, this juice satisfies on multiple levels. It combines the rooty sweetness of carrot with the zing of ginger, spice of cayenne, and the balance of lime.

7 medium carrots
1 inch fresh gingerroot, peeled
¼ cup cilantro
½ medium lime, peeled
Juice.

Top with a pinch of cayenne pepper and pinch of pink Himalayan salt.

JUICY TIP

A pinch of pink Himalayan salt in a bottle of filtered water is extra hydrating to the body on a hot day. If Himalayan salt is not available in a store near you, it can be easily sourced from online purveyors.

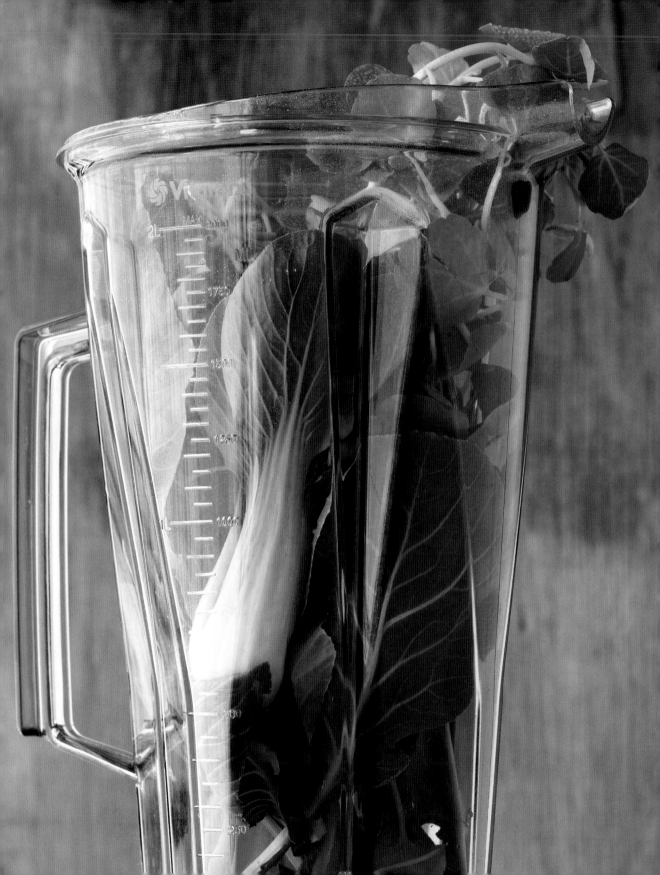

ULTRA WELLNESS AND SUPERFOODS

By this part of the Green Curve, turning a handful of fresh ingredients into luscious blended drinks has become second nature. In Phase 3, we encourage you to strut your smoothie skills by expanding your ingredient repertoire to include even more diverse raw ingredients as well as delectable, homemade nut milk and supercharged superfoods. The smoothie becomes a true meal-in-a-cup, enhanced with healthy fats and proteins like nut butters, avocado, coconut meat, hemp or chia seeds, or given a green boost with spirulina. You can give your blended drinks a great chocolate flavor by adding nutrient-packed raw cacao and the tonic-herb maca root, or infuse your smoothie with extra antioxidants via a handful of scarlet goji berries. As always, use the following recipes as a starting-off point, a place from which you can freestyle as you get to know new ingredients and experiment in different ways with familiar ones.

NUT MILK

A few steps are all it takes to make a liquid food that—quite frankly—completely outshines the store-bought, packaged kind. Light, fresh, mildly sweet, and actually tasting of the real food it's made from.

Making nut milk involves soaking raw nuts to neutralize the enzyme inhibitors that naturally occur in nuts, meaning they become much more digestible. (Allergic to nuts? Try our hemp milk recipe variation.)

High-speed blender. A Vitamix or Blendtec is the most efficient option; a regular blender may also work depending on its strength. A masticating juicer can also be used (with its low RPMs, some say this preserves more nutrients).

Nut milk bag, available at health food stores. Another option is to use a piece of cheesecloth inside a metal strainer, though you may need to double the cloth to ensure that tiny nut pieces don't sneak through.

Medium-size mixing bowl or measuring jug to catch the nut milk.

Glass jar with lid to store the nut milk.

Raw nuts. The easiest and most cost-effective nut milk to make is almond milk. Always look for raw almonds—roasted will not work.

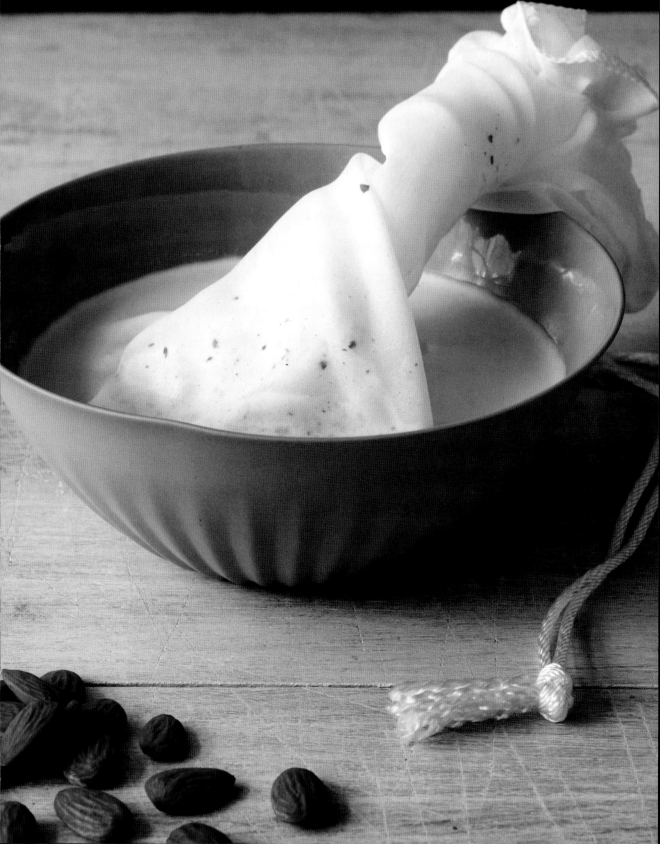

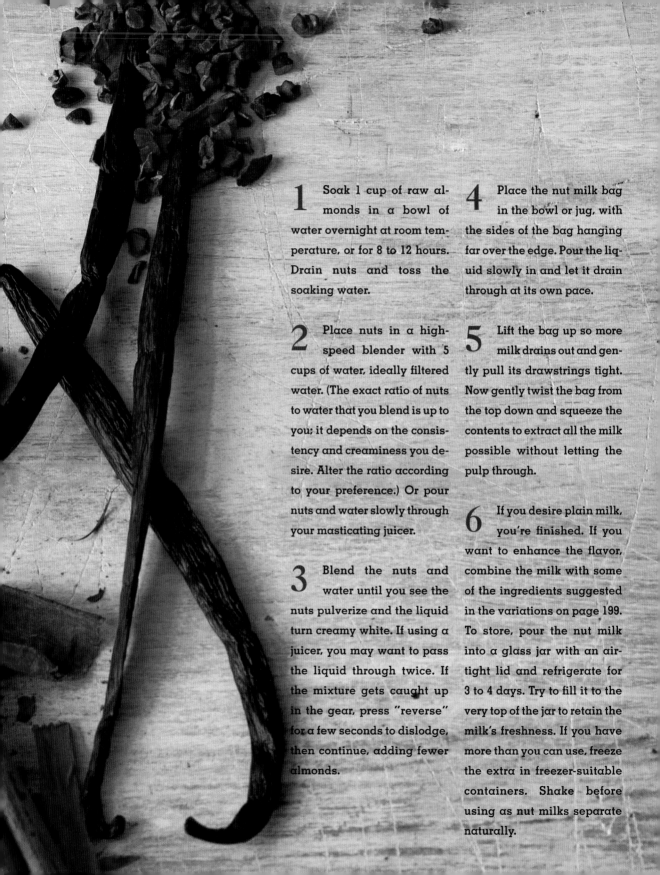

1 Soak 1 cup of raw almonds in a bowl of water overnight at room temperature, or for 8 to 12 hours. Drain nuts and toss the soaking water.

2 Place nuts in a high-speed blender with 5 cups of water, ideally filtered water. (The exact ratio of nuts to water that you blend is up to you; it depends on the consistency and creaminess you desire. Alter the ratio according to your preference.) Or pour nuts and water slowly through your masticating juicer.

3 Blend the nuts and water until you see the nuts pulverize and the liquid turn creamy white. If using a juicer, you may want to pass the liquid through twice. If the mixture gets caught up in the gear, press "reverse" for a few seconds to dislodge, then continue, adding fewer almonds.

4 Place the nut milk bag in the bowl or jug, with the sides of the bag hanging far over the edge. Pour the liquid slowly in and let it drain through at its own pace.

5 Lift the bag up so more milk drains out and gently pull its drawstrings tight. Now gently twist the bag from the top down and squeeze the contents to extract all the milk possible without letting the pulp through.

6 If you desire plain milk, you're finished. If you want to enhance the flavor, combine the milk with some of the ingredients suggested in the variations on page 199. To store, pour the nut milk into a glass jar with an airtight lid and refrigerate for 3 to 4 days. Try to fill it to the very top of the jar to retain the milk's freshness. If you have more than you can use, freeze the extra in freezer-suitable containers. Shake before using as nut milks separate naturally.

Irresistible Brazil Nut Milk

Follow directions on page 198 using 1 cup Brazil nuts and 5 cups water (adjust the ratio depending on the thickness desired), but do not soak the Brazil nuts. Blend with dates, pinch of sea salt or pink Himalayan salt, and vanilla bean or vanilla essence to taste.

Vanilla Almond Milk

Pour almond milk into blender with ½ to 1 vanilla beans (or a dash of vanilla essence), filtered water, and dates to taste. Advanced level: Add a pinch of turmeric for a golden-yellow, extrahealing drink!

Cinnamon Cashew Milk

Follow directions on page 198 using 1 cup cashews and 5 cups water (adjust the ratio depending on the thickness desired), but soak the cashews only for 2 to 2½ hours. Blend with dates, pinch of sea salt or pink Himalayan salt, vanilla bean or vanilla essence, cinnamon.

Chai Hemp Milk

Follow directions on page 198 using 1 cup hemp seeds and 5 cups water (adjust the ratio depending on the thickness desired), but do not soak the hemp seeds. Blend with a nub of fresh ginger diced small, a dash of cinnamon, seeds from 2 to 3 pods of cardamom, dates to taste.

JUICY TIP

The most commonly available almonds that are labeled "raw" have actually been pasteurized using steam or even chemicals, or possibly irradiated, though they have not been roasted at high heat. It is not easy to find 100 percent unpasteurized nuts, though they may be available at farmers' markets and from online sources. Their price is significantly higher—the same goes for truly "raw" nut butters—though fans say that the taste and benefits are, too. Buying organic almonds labeled "raw" will ensure your nuts didn't undergo a chemical pasteurization process.

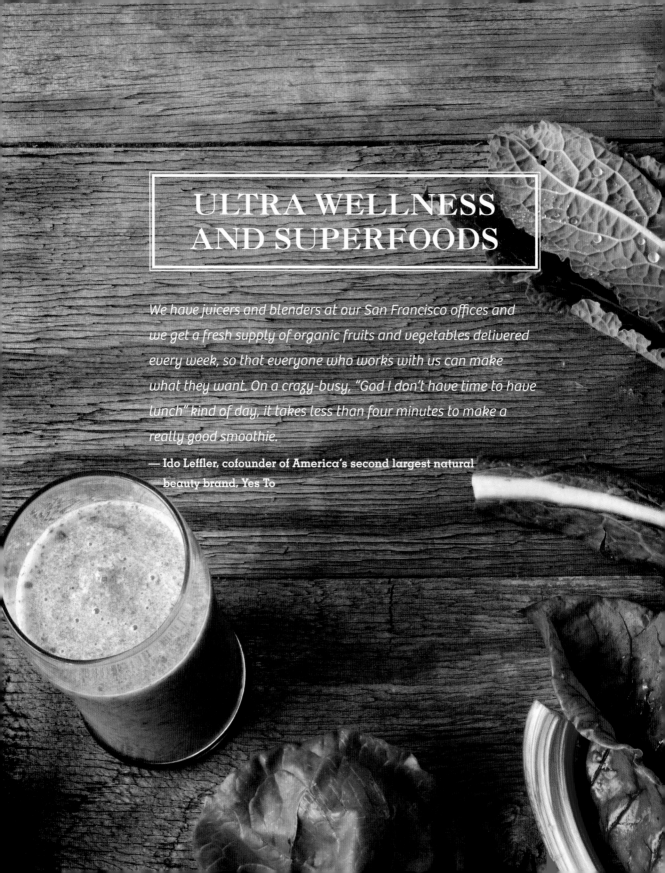

ULTRA WELLNESS
AND SUPERFOODS

*We have juicers and blenders at our San Francisco offices and
we get a fresh supply of organic fruits and vegetables delivered
every week, so that everyone who works with us can make
what they want. On a crazy-busy, "God I don't have time to have
lunch" kind of day, it takes less than four minutes to make a
really good smoothie.*

— Ido Leffler, cofounder of America's second largest natural
   beauty brand, Yes To

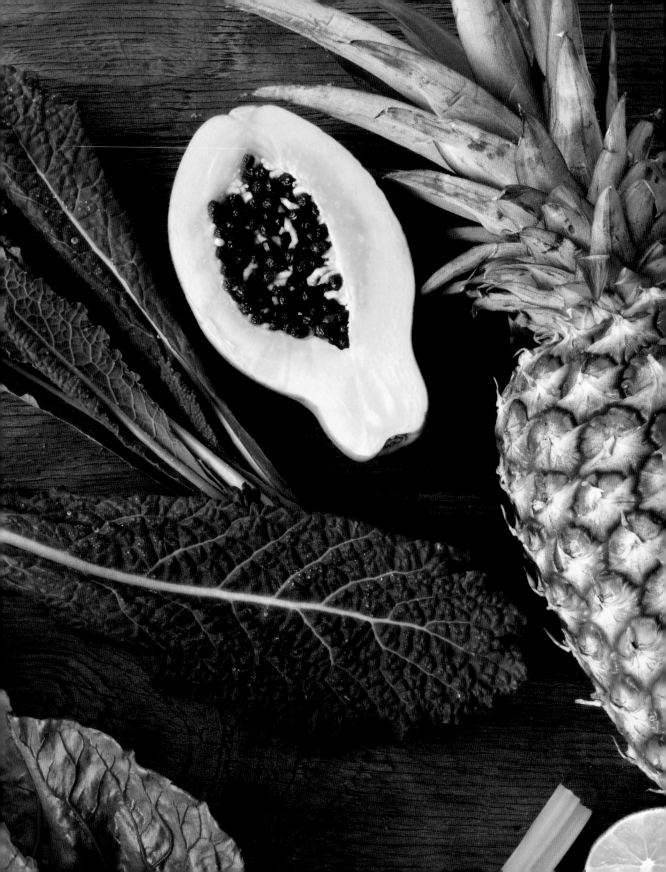

Hero's Garden

Go ultragreen in a flash by mixing four kinds of green in a single cup. Two phenomenal green leaves blend with tart, green apple and the lush texture of avocado. (Play with the amount of avocado to alter the creaminess.) Make your own apple juice before blending—an extra step that reaps big flavor rewards.

2 leaves Swiss chard
1 cup kale
½ medium green apple
½ medium avocado
1 cup fresh apple juice
Blend.

Optional: Use water instead of apple juice.

Antioxidant All-Star

Dial up the flavor, color, and goodness as a trio of irresistible colors—red, blue, and purple—combine with three super-green leaves in a drink that infuses you with disease-preventing antioxidants. Red pomegranate pops with tart flavor, blueberries balance them with sweetness, and acaí deepens the effect with its purple, cherry-berry taste.

1 pack frozen acaí
¼ cup pomegranate seeds
½ cup blueberries
2 leaves Swiss chard
2 leaves collard greens
1 cup kale
½ medium green apple
1 cup filtered water
Blend.

Emerald Escape

Though tough-textured collards are typically eaten braised with broth, blending breaks down the cell walls effectively too, releasing the prized nutrition. Think: carotenoids, vitamin K, vitamin C, vitamin E, folate, and manganese. Here, collard juice is transformed into an energizing elixir that's sweet and savory when combined with pineapple, lime, cilantro, and an energizing hit of blue-green spirulina—a nourishing plant-food from earth's clean waters.

2 leaves collard greens
1 cup papaya
1 cup pineapple
¼ cup cilantro
½ tablespoon spirulina powder
1 cup fresh coconut water
½ medium lime, peeled
Blend.

Optional: Sweeten smoothie with 1 to 2 dates, if needed.

Island Blue

The aquabotanical called AFA blue-green algae is considered by many to be a wonder food. Sourced from deep, remote lakes, it is the wild-harvested counterpart to spirulina, and considered by many to have superior nutritional quality; it energizes, focuses, and balances the mind and body and delivers resilience to stress. Coconut water works in synergy, helping the body absorb more of the algae's omega-3s.

1 freshly cracked young Thai coconut, water and meat
1 ounce blue green algae
Blend.

SPIRULINA

Spirulina has been on earth since the dawn of time. This blue-green algae grows wild in freshwater lakes and waterways and is cultivated for nutritional use primarily in Hawaii. Its intense color is made up of green chlorophyll and blue phycocyanin, a health-promoting pigment. Spirulina lovers say the algae's highly absorbable, complete protein gives them a boost—vegan athletes often use it in their dietary regimes. In addition, its broad-spectrum nutrients, including essential gamma-linoleic acid, maintains a healthy nervous system. Spirulina's flavor is unusual and a little lakelike, so start very small and let your palate adjust!

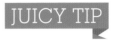

JUICY TIP

Notoriously tricky to open without spattering your clothes and counters, a pomegranate can be tamed by first slicing off the top to reveal the seeds, then scoring it lengthwise into six sections with a paring knife. Carefully split the sections apart, peel off the white pith, crack into smaller segments if necessary, and pop the seeds into a bowl. If this is too messy, submerge the fruit in a bowl of water to split and scoop.

In our stores we use E3Live, an organic, wild-gathered blue-green algae from Upper Klamath Lake, Oregon; it's a fresh frozen pulp that is thawed before using. Start slowly due to its detoxifying effect. Always be sure your algae superfoods come from reputable sources.

Juice Smarts: Reputed to have helped Taoist wise men live for centuries, the goji berry is part food, part medicine. Normally purchased in their dried form, good-quality goji berries should be slightly moist, not brittle or very dull in color. Because they're usually imported from overseas, it's wise to research your brands if you want to ensure chemical-free berries. Some farmers' markets now have locally grown fresh berries. Mix a handful of gojis with raw cacao nibs and nuts for a superb on-the-go snack.

The Sage's Smoothie

Go wild for the goji berry, the tiny, flame-red superfruit famed in China and Tibet for its longevity-boosting properties and cherished by foodies for its delicious, cranberry-cherry taste. Add a boost of chia seeds—long used by native Americans of the Southwest for endurance and hydration—to nourishing coconut for a hearty drink that will tide you over for hours.

1 freshly cracked young Thai coconut, meat and water
½ cup papaya
2 tablespoons soaked goji berries
1 tablespoon chia seeds
½ cup parsley
½ medium frozen banana
3 dates, pitted
Blend.

Soak chia seeds in the blender liquid for 10 minutes before blending so they absorb liquid. This helps them to hydrate you more effectively.

Lynsey's Joyful Almond

This rich and creamy smoothie can satisfy your sweet tooth when you're craving a dessert, or fuel you through a rigorous morning with its slow-burning fats. For a pop of pleasurable texture, use crunchy, raw cacao nibs instead of powder.

1 cup almond milk
2 tablespoons almond butter
½ tablespoon raw cacao
¼ cup frozen coconut milk
½ medium banana
2 dates, pitted
Blend.

As a winter athlete, my focus is on warmth, protein that can last all day when I'm in the mountains, good fats, and hydration—it is important in helping to avoid altitude fatigue and to support brain function and circulation. I believe in filling my cup with substance, whether I'm shooting a ski film in Alaska or having a long day of meetings or travel for SheJumps, the girls' empowerment organization I cofounded. Even in the most unusual locations, it is easy to fill a blender, press a button and go—I feel 100 percent more confident when I've been able to take care of my nutrition myself, and not have to depend on what's provided.

—Lynsey Dyer, professional big mountain skier

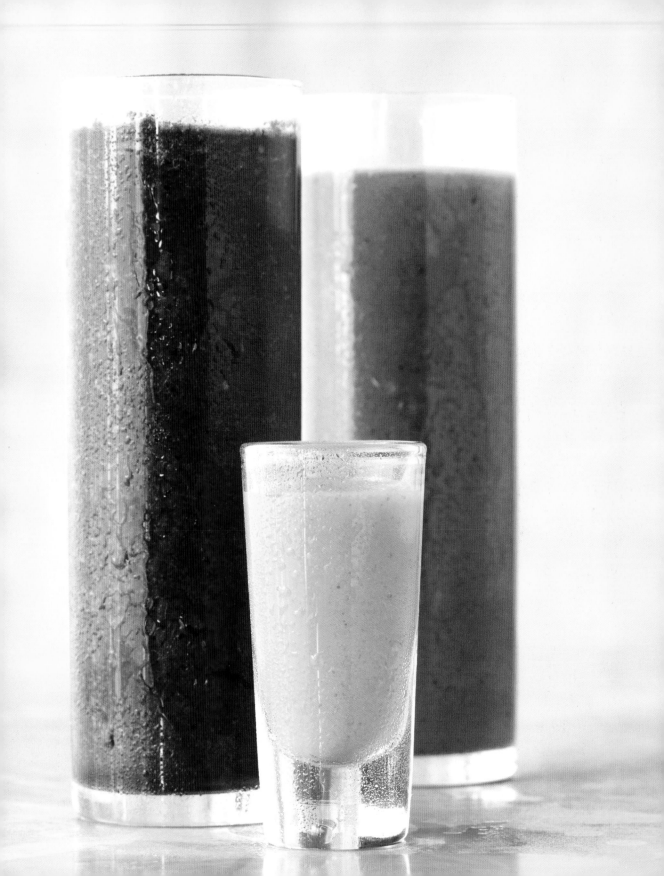

THE NEXT
FRUIT FRONTIER

Stumbling upon the next hot sensation from the fruit world makes the art of smoothies extra enticing. At Juice Generation we are certifiable flavor hunters—always searching for the next fruity frontier, motivated by the hunger for a new experience of flavor, color, and texture. Meet our three favorite little-known fruits with the power to seduce body, mind, and senses.

ARONIA BERRIES

Watch out acaí, there's a new superberry in town—and it's native to North America. The aronia berry's violet-black flesh is virtually exploding with antioxidant power and antidiabetic and anticancer effects. The tart, slightly sour flavor gives it a menacing alias—black chokeberry—but balance it out with complementary ingredients and you get a delectable dose of ultrawellness that is sourced on U.S. soil. Aronia berries are still new players in the natural-foods market. Frozen packs and powdered fruit are available online or ask your local health-food store to consider supplying them from one of the new crop of North American suppliers. If not available, substitute acaí.

All-Star Aronia

½ cup aronia berries
½ cup strawberries
1 cup spinach
½ medium frozen banana
1 cup fresh apple juice
Blend.

Pink Pitaya

1 freshly cracked young Thai coconut, water and meat
1 cup pitaya
½ medium banana
Blend.

Buckthorn Blast

1 ounce sea buckthorn puree
1 ounce filtered water
Blend.

PITAYA

This diva of fruits—also known as dragonfruit—has a hot-pink outside that conjures a feathered bird of paradise and reveals white, or sometimes vibrant fuchsia, flesh inside that's graphically studded with tiny black seeds. Its delicate flavor, reminiscent of a pear crossed with a kiwi and a melon, has a refreshing and subtle effect that does best when paired with equally mild flavors. Typically sold at Asian food markets, the pitaya is ripe when the leafy scales on the outside are slightly dry and shriveled, not hard and green. Simply slice the fruit in half and scoop the flesh and seeds out with a spoon.

SEA BUCKTHORN BERRIES

Traditionally plucked from shrubs high in the Himalayas, the bright-orange sea buckthorn berry has been used since ancient times in Asian healing and is poised to become the next goji berry. Westerners are discovering why this tangy fruit is nature's ultra multivitamin—in addition to a cocktail of 190 bioactive nutrients, it contains the hard-to-find omega-7, a fatty acid said to support healthy intestines, weight levels, and cardiovascular health as well as keep skin, hair, and nails at their best. Sea buckthorn is currently most easily acquired as a prebottled liquid supplement or as capsule supplements. In the future, it may become possible to find the fruit as a frozen puree.

MACA & MORE: SUPER BOOSTERS

Treat your body like a temple by integrating a pair of nature's most nourishing plant foods into your daily drinks. These two ingredients have been used—and revered—by people in far-flung locales for millennia for their strengthening, energizing, and balancing properties. But only recently have they entered our modern-day pantries under the tag line of superfood—eatables that have an exceptional amount of wellness-enhancing qualities housed in one turbo-charged package.

RAW CACAO

Solids from the cacao bean that are usually cooked to make chocolate candy bars, but that lose many of their beneficial properties when roasted—can be added to a smoothie as raw cocoa powder or crunchy cacao nibs for a hearty boost of antioxidants, iron, and magnesium.

MACA ROOT

An Andean tuber that has a faintly golden-malted taste—is available as a powder to sprinkle into all kinds of juices and smoothies—delivering a gentle boost in alertness and a handful of significant health benefits.

JUICY TIP

Cacao taken in large amounts can make some people feel "wired" and overstimulated, so it is still important to tune in to your body's response to evaluate how it works for you and in what quantity. Seek out 100 percent raw, organic cacao products. A Fair Trade stamp on the package helps you know it's ethically sourced from overseas communities.

These pick-me-uppers can replace the lift of morning caffeine for some people, without the edgy side effects and with lots of extra benefits: Cacao has been called the "food of the gods" for its phenomenal combination of compounds that nourish the body, increase alertness and, thanks to the "bliss chemical" anandamide as well as tryptophan and serotonin, noticeably raise the mood. (Plus, science is now showing how these compounds help protect us from a myriad of modern-day problems like cardiovascular disease and type 2 diabetes.) Maca, used as a daily staple food by high-altitude mountain dwellers in Bolivia and Peru, is a famed adaptogen—a tonic herb that strengthens the body against stress and delivers endurance, as well as reproductive health and virility! What's not to enjoy about this superduo of superfoods?

Maca root powder is easy to find in most natural foods stores. It also goes wonderfully with nut milks spiked with cacao and vanilla.

Juice Smarts: A raw-foods chef's secret weapon, Irish moss is a seaweed that delivers a luscious, creamy texture to smoothies and desserts without the caloric boost of nuts and seeds, and with important iodine and iron, as well as antioxidants. (Carrageenan, used in boxed nondairy milks, is its processed and concentrated extract.) The authentic, whole-food ingredient is a cold-water seaweed harvested off the coast of Ireland and that should come fully dried—as always, check the source and quality of your purchase—and it can turn an everyday drink, as well as a thick blended dessert or creamy pie, into an out-of-this-world experience. Soak it for about 20 minutes in water to rehydrate before blending.

Maca Master

History tells us that Incan warriors used maca for fortitude and courage before heading into battle; it's not surprising that this South American root is a go-to superfood helping us stay focused and fearless in the fast-lane of contemporary life. And it won't spark gustatory trepidation: Its slightly malty aroma evokes a malt ball or graham cracker.

1 pack frozen acaí
1 cup strawberries
1 tablespoon maca root
   powder
½ medium banana
1 cup fresh coconut water
3 dates, pitted
Blend.

Hack That Smoothie! Add a tablespoon of soaked chia seeds to give an extra hit of nutrition and hydration to your super drink.

Queen of Fruits

Blending two of the original superfruits—the dark-red (read: antioxidant-filled) pomegranate with the delicate, white-fleshed mangosteen—this smoothie delivers a medley of surprisingly enchanting, tart-sweet tastes. Mangosteen, the official national fruit of Thailand that is famed for its aromatic flavor, has long been nicknamed the "queen of fruits" by tropical fruit lovers.

2 medium mangosteens,
   peeled and pitted
1 medium kiwi, pitted
1 cup fresh pomegranate juice
1 inch fresh gingerroot, peeled
3 dates, pitted
Blend.

Hack That Smoothie! Add a handful of mild green leaves like spinach.

Drink of the Gods

Indulge the senses in the luxuriant experience of chocolate and hemp milk, made creamier with the addition of an unusual natural thickener—a seaweed that secretly adds more minerals to your drink.

1 cup hemp milk
1 tablespoon raw cacao
¼ cup soaked Irish moss
1 tablespoon coconut oil
½ medium banana
3 dates, pitted
Blend.

Juice cleanses are the perfect way to get back on track after you've had a weekend full of consecutive pig-out sessions. They're also just an easy, great way to do something healthy for your body. I'm a big fan of all fruit juices, so I love juice with pear, or watermelon lime, or a spicy lemonade. But I also know that vegetables rule and are the best for you, so when it's time to get hardcore, I drink a green juice with a veggie like kale. But those are the most difficult ones for me, so give me a green juice with something sweet like apple and a little lemon and I can almost pretend it's dessert!

—Gayle King, coanchor of *CBS This Morning* and editor at large of *O, The Oprah Magazine*

CLEANSE AND REVIVE

USING YOUR JUICING TOOLS FOR DETOXING AND HEALING

The three phases of juices and smoothies may have delivered all kinds of results—from enjoying a new awareness of food, to feeling confident in the kitchen with new health-giving ingredients, to noticing a higher energy level, clearer mind, better-functioning body, and more glowing skin. The more your new tools become habitual, the easier it will be to continue to refresh, restore, and energize yourself, on your own terms. Reaching the top of the Green Curve is just the beginning of a new way of being, in which it feels second nature to reach for vital greens and whole-food ingredients to take care of yourself wisely, day in and day out.

Taking good care of yourself may also involve occasionally doing short and easy juice cleanses or using the power of juice to fight colds and other illnesses.

THE RESET

At Juice Generation we think of cleanses like short resets for your body. They are dietary programs featuring a customized mix of fresh juices, coconut water, and nut or seed milks (if you choose) that you follow for one or a few days to give your digestive system a break and flood your cells with rejuvenating, lifting, and clearing energy. Doing one day of liquid-only foods, or as much as three days in a row, can be a simple and easy-to-succeed way to come back to balance in body, mind, and spirit, without overhauling your entire life to do it.

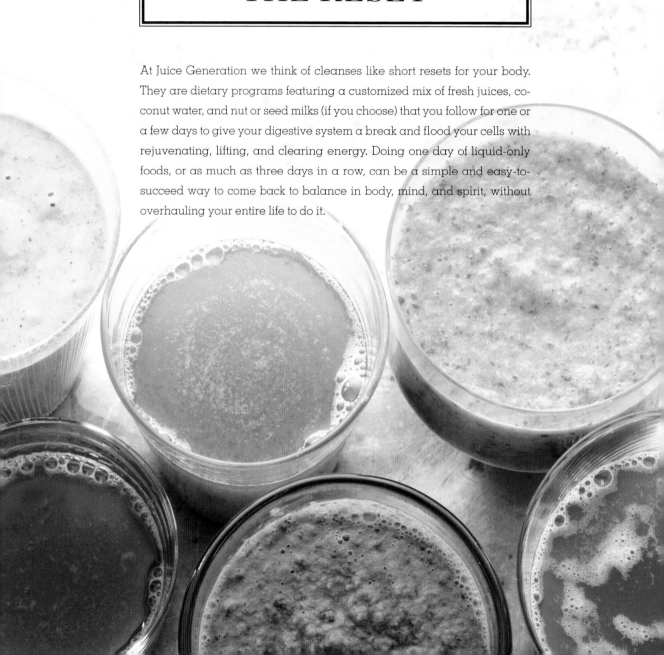

At Juice Generation, we call these little breaks from regular food programming *resets* because they are short programs that aren't aiming too high—they're not trying to reverse decades-worth of toxins in 24 or 72 hours. Their goal is not to shed weight or heal chronic health issues. (Those goals can be addressed through a long-term plan of smart nutrition and strategic cleansing programs—but you'll want to accomplish this slowly and over time, and ideally with the guidance of a good practitioner or health coach. For reference, our signature Cooler Cleanse juice deliveries offer six juices that provide approximately 1,200 calories in a day.)

These smaller, shorter programs of one, two, or three days on juice-only diets are about finding your equilibrium and coming back to center; unplugging from ordinary eating and drinking habits; resting your system and boosting immunity; and alkalinizing your blood and feeling a rebound in energy, lightness, and clarity as a result. You are giving your essential detoxification organs a lift by adding lots of natural antioxidants that bind to toxins and convert them to harmless substances and nutrients, such as beta-carotene, that help the liver do its work. This is a key to successful preventive health care.

A cleanse can also reset your relationship to food. It's human nature to fall into food routines that don't support us fully, whether it's consuming foods and drinks that irritate our systems, that fatigue us rather than fuel us, or that don't have enough vital force of live enzymes and micronutrients to help our bodies do their best work. Or, we might already have a balanced, smart diet, but in the busyness of life, that good food gets consumed in unconscious and rushed ways—something that all healers say compromises digestion and overall well-being.

Cleansing programs don't suit everyone, so there's no need to make it a priority if it does not feel right for your body. But for many people, taking a break from regular eating habits can give fresh perspective on what and how we eat daily, helping us to *see and feel* what works and what does not, and motivating a positive shift toward a cleaner, greener, happier, and healthier way of being for the longer term.

THE GREEN CURVE CLEANSE

After spending time on the Green Curve, you've probably already experienced some changes in what you crave and what you consume each day. You might have seen some of your existing food habits with fresh, new eyes. Simply implementing daily green drinks into your diet is in itself a mild and steady cleanse: You are slowly and steadily replacing unhealthy foods with healthy ones; you're feeding the liver, the intestines, and the bloodstream with trace nutrients they may previously have lacked; and over time, by replacing sugary foods and foods that may have been irritating you, like gluten and pasteurized dairy, you are allowing the environment of your intestines to rebalance and repair itself. In other words, you've been doing a mild daily cleansing program every day!

It's so stressful during fashion show preparation time that you end up kind of eating all sorts of crazy things. And you're at the studio until three in the morning. So it's great once the show is done to be able to do a cleanse and get back on track. It's like we've repaired ourselves from all the damage that show week has done to our bodies.

—**Peter Som, fashion designer**

At Juice Generation, we recommend that those new to cleansing programs try a 1-Day or a 3-Day Juice Cleanse, depending on their goals. Some people then go on to try a 5-Day Cleanse at a later date. This longer cleanse is best with a little more preparation and, often, some oversight from a health coach or advisor. All juice cleanse programs have the potential to create uncomfortable detoxification symptoms—though if you have already cleaned up your diet and been using green drinks regularly, you will likely experience much less of this effect. Longer cleansing programs require extra care to ensure your system is getting the best support. Here, we introduce you to the two shorter versions of juice cleansing.

Juice Smarts: Why no smoothies? Cleansing and detoxification programs use juices, including coconut waters and nut milks, but not smoothies, because the fiber-free juices and drinks are absorbed with minimal work by your digestive system, freeing up the most energy possible for your body to put toward detoxification and healing.

JUICE FOR A DAY

WHEN TO DO IT

You've overindulged in food and drink and feel the consequences, and want a day to reset your system; you want to take a quiet day oriented toward rest and rejuvenation, to give your digestive system a rest and help support your detoxification system, as part of a greater goal of balance and well-being.

WHAT TO DO

Over your day, consume six fresh-made juices including coconut water and nut or seed milks, if you desire, at regular intervals (approximately every two hours) in lieu of your regular meals and snacks. Include a spectrum of juices with a good selection of green drinks for maximum benefit, as greens have the most nutrients to support the detoxification system. We include juice suggestions here, but you can also customize it yourself. However, do not consume six fruit-based and root-based (i.e., carrot and beet) drinks, as this is an overload of sugar. Mix it up and *lean into the green*. Most people prefer to have a nut milk as the final drink of the day, as the fats and protein gently nourish through the night and also help bind to toxins that may be have been released, facilitating their excretion. Starting the day with hot water and lemon and ending it with a warm, herbal tea is especially helpful. Have your drinks at room temperature, not ice cold, and sip them slowly.

If you need more than six juices to get by, add another—make it a nut milk if you want extra calories. Keep all your juices clean and simple without adding in fats (like coconut oil or avocado). Drink plenty of water throughout the day; herbal teas are fine, but try to cut the caffeine. If you must, have lightly steeped green tea.

Try to avoid snacks! If you're struggling with hunger, a small piece of fruit plus raw nuts or nut butter may help.

If possible, rest well on this day. Get to bed early. Take the time for you.

One option for the Juice-for-a-Day program is to begin your cleanse at dinner time the night before, so that your first juice is at night. The next day, continue with your next five juices, and at dinnertime ease out of the cleanse with a light meal such as soup, salad, steamed vegetables.

MAKE YOUR OWN PROGRAM

A wise cleansing menu comprises a spectrum of drinks that focus on low-fruit greens. There is no one way to write a program of six juices in one day, but an ideal day could include a morning green drink; a midmorning drink featuring grapefruit; a vegetable-rich green drink midday or a nut milk for more nourishment; a coconut water or green drink in the midafternoon; a fruit or vegetable juice in the late afternoon, and a nut milk for soothing nourishment in the evening.

For the optimal experience, choose from the following recipes: 2 to 3 dark green juices, 1 to 2 lighter green or fruit-based juices, 1 to 2 nut milks, and 1 coconut water, for a total of six drinks in each 24-hour period (or more if you are very hungry).

WHAT YOU MIGHT EXPERIENCE

This is a simple reset that helps to clear the mental and physical fog or reinvigorate your senses and allow for rest and recharging.

HOW TO USE IT

Use it as an occasional tool; or do it once a week for three or four weeks in a row to experience and integrate gentle self-care into your life in a meaningful way. Some people like to do a Juice-for-a-Day reset once a week, for example on a Sunday, as part of a plan for greater well-being.

THE 3-DAY CLEANSE

WHEN TO DO IT

You want to do a deeper dive into refreshing and boosting your body, and have some extra time to take care of yourself, rest well, and cut back on busy demands; you are feeling weighed down, sluggish, or off-track, and want to do a significant jump-start toward higher health and wellness.

WHAT TO DO

It is wise to plan the 3-Day Cleanse with some foresight. The two or three days before and after the cleanse are an opportunity to "ease in" and "ease out" of your cleanse by consuming clean, freshly prepared foods free of irritating effects. This means a fairly simple diet based on lightly cooked vegetables, soups, and broths, easily digestible proteins cooked simply, and no common irritants like gluten, dairy, and eggs, as well as processed or heavy foods, excessive sweets, alcohol, and strong caffeine. Do not use these pre- and post-days to cut back on calories; the idea is to take care of yourself kindly.

By easing in and easing out of your cleanse in this way, you'll give your body the maximum nutritional and energetic benefits by taking a load off the digestive system and removing any irritating factors, so that more energy can go toward detoxification and healing. You'll feel, and look, more refreshed and you will sleep better as a result.

———

On each day of the cleanse, follow the What to Do directions for the 1-Day Cleanse and pick your drinks according to the What to Drink list.

In addition, you'll want to keep these points in mind:

Try to get to bed early. Light exercise is recommended as movement stimulates the lymphatic system to move waste products out of the body. But hard workouts that use significant calories and require recovery are best left for before and after your cleanse. Turn off your phone and read a book instead.

During the 3-Day Cleanse, it is ideal to support your elimination system to ensure that the body's naturally produced toxins, as well as any not natural toxins that may be released, can leave your system efficiently.

Over these days, you will help yourself get best benefits if you:

■ Breathe deeply; time on the yoga mat is very well spent.

■ Ensure that you have good bowel movements every day, which can be helped with a non-stimulating supplement like magnesium powder before bed.

■ Sweat in a sauna if you can; or do a short, sweaty workout that is not too demanding.

Many people find the first day slightly challenging. Many feel no unsettling side effects, but it's possible to feel some symptoms of withdrawal from caffeine, as well as symptoms of detoxification, which can range from headaches to fatigue to irritation. Try not to see these as wrong, but rather as symptoms of something clearing out. They'll pass.

WHAT YOU MIGHT EXPERIENCE

By the end of the three days, you may feel lighter, brighter, clearer in mind and body. You may feel renewed energy and focus and notice your eyes, skin, and hair looking more vital. You may have a new sensitivity to how the foods you eat either make you feel uplifted—or make you tired. You may have lost a few pounds, but remember, this is not the goal of the cleanse.

HOW TO USE IT

This short reset can be used on a periodic basis, such as every season or every few months. It is important to always remember that juice cleanses are kick starts for healthy, long-term habits and resting periods to recharge and refresh; they are not quick fixes for neglecting your well-being or substitutes for a smart, longer-term strategy.

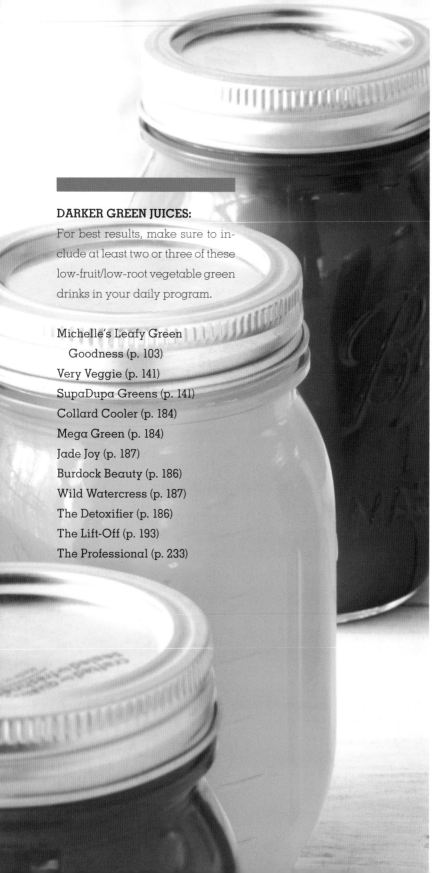

DARKER GREEN JUICES:

For best results, make sure to include at least two or three of these low-fruit/low-root vegetable green drinks in your daily program.

Michelle's Leafy Green
   Goodness (p. 103)
Very Veggie (p. 141)
SupaDupa Greens (p. 141)
Collard Cooler (p. 184)
Mega Green (p. 184)
Jade Joy (p. 187)
Burdock Beauty (p. 186)
Wild Watercress (p. 187)
The Detoxifier (p. 186)
The Lift-Off (p. 193)
The Professional (p. 233)

LIGHTER GREEN JUICES:

As these contain slightly more fruits or roots, it's ideal to include these in moderation: just one or two in your daily program.

Debra's Green Elixir (p. 93)
Hail to Kale (p. 103)
Very Veggie (p. 141)
Get Ur Green On (p. 141)
Blake's Intoxicating
   Detoxification (p. 144)
Golden Goddess (p. 190)
Salsa Samba (p. 193)
Michael's Go-to Greens (p. 225)
Gaia's Garden (p. 233)
Verdant Vista (p. 233)

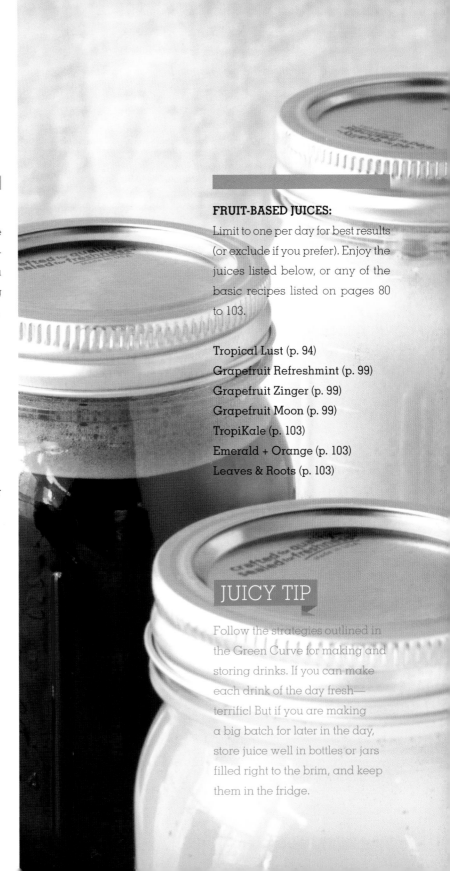

NUT MILKS:

It's recommended that you have at least one nut milk a day, consumed at the end of the day if you like. Add a second nut milk during the day if you feel a lot of hunger.

Vanilla Almond Milk (p. 199)
Irresistible Brazil Nut
   Milk (p. 199)
Cinnamon Cashew Milk (p. 199)
Chai Hemp Milk (p. 199)

COCONUT WATER

Have one optional coconut water a day for refreshment.

Plain coconut water from a fresh-cracked nut

Island Blue (p. 203)

FRUIT-BASED JUICES:

Limit to one per day for best results (or exclude if you prefer). Enjoy the juices listed below, or any of the basic recipes listed on pages 80 to 103.

Tropical Lust (p. 94)
Grapefruit Refreshmint (p. 99)
Grapefruit Zinger (p. 99)
Grapefruit Moon (p. 99)
TropiKale (p. 103)
Emerald + Orange (p. 103)
Leaves & Roots (p. 103)

JUICY TIP

Follow the strategies outlined in the Green Curve for making and storing drinks. If you can make each drink of the day fresh— terrific! But if you are making a big batch for later in the day, store juice well in bottles or jars filled right to the brim, and keep them in the fridge.

JUICE FARMACY

We first developed juice remedies for the Broadway performers who frequent our 9th Avenue store. They requested ginger-spiked elixirs to help counteract a cold or a warm, throat-soothing concoction that wouldn't dehydrate the vocal chords like caffeine does—all so that the show could go on. These actors, singers, and dancers are unusually attuned to what supports and sustains the body. By requesting these healing concoctions, they showed us how a medicine kit of juices, hot drinks, and juice shots can help anyone find their way back to show-stopping form.

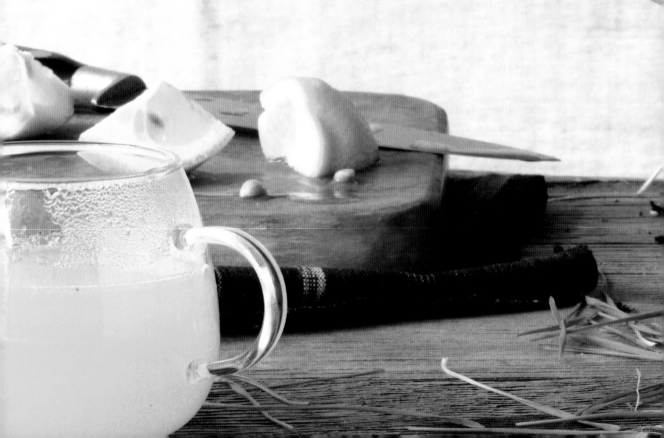

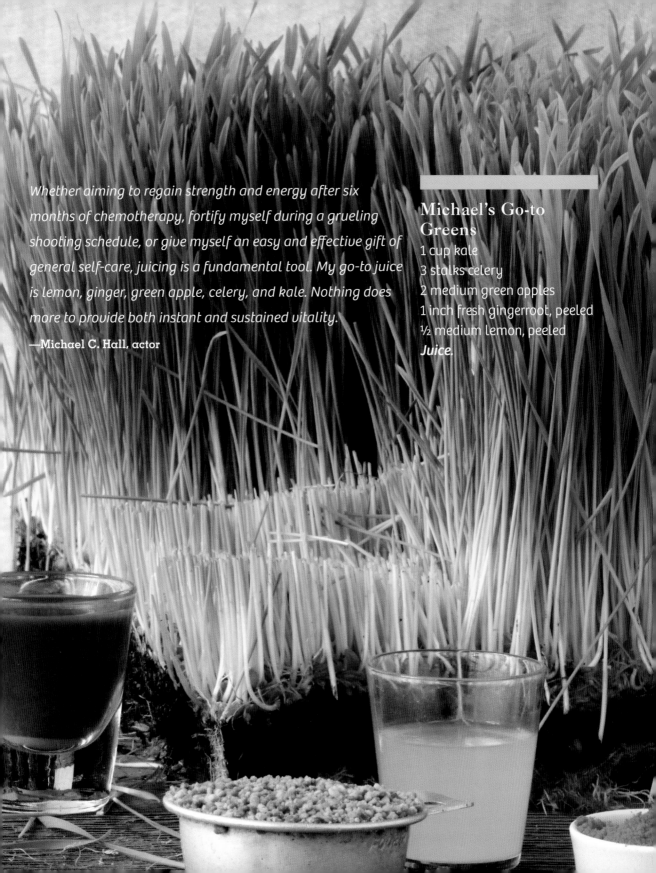

Whether aiming to regain strength and energy after six months of chemotherapy, fortify myself during a grueling shooting schedule, or give myself an easy and effective gift of general self-care, juicing is a fundamental tool. My go-to juice is lemon, ginger, green apple, celery, and kale. Nothing does more to provide both instant and sustained vitality.

—**Michael C. Hall**, actor

Michael's Go-to Greens

1 cup kale
3 stalks celery
2 medium green apples
1 inch fresh gingerroot, peeled
½ medium lemon, peeled

Juice.

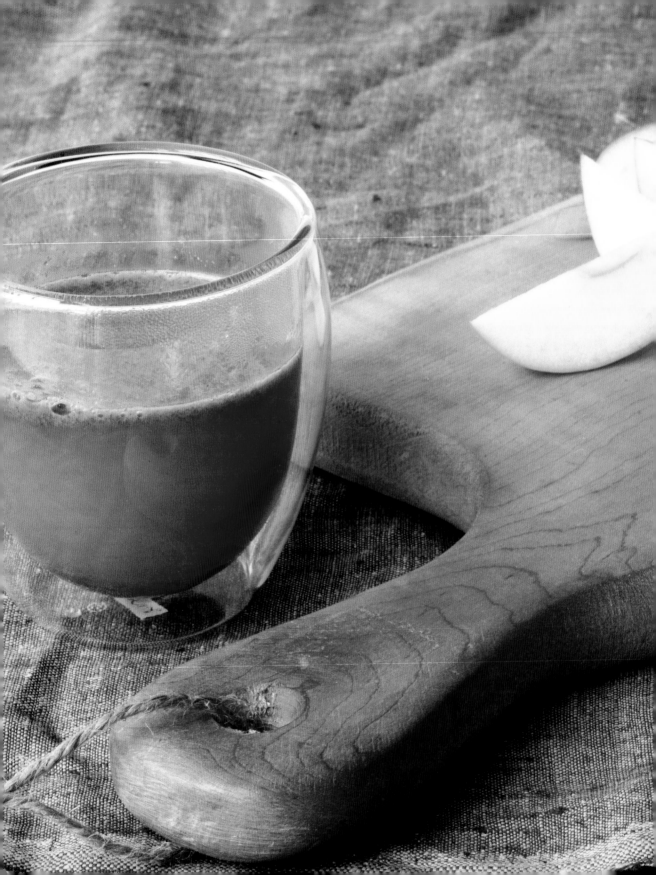

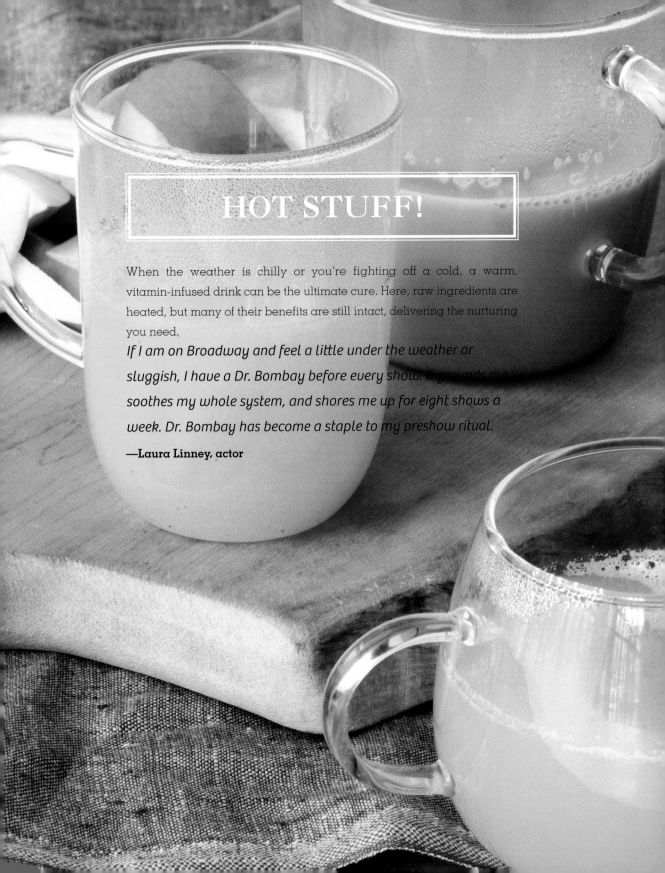

HOT STUFF!

When the weather is chilly or you're fighting off a cold, a warm, vitamin-infused drink can be the ultimate cure. Here, raw ingredients are heated, but many of their benefits are still intact, delivering the nurturing you need.

If I am on Broadway and feel a little under the weather or sluggish, I have a Dr. Bombay before every show. It grounds me, soothes my whole system, and shores me up for eight shows a week. Dr. Bombay has become a staple to my preshow ritual.

—Laura Linney, actor

Cold Warrior

Zinc and echinacea are prized for their sniffle-fighting capabilities. A few drops of these liquid supplements give a tasty warming brew a healing bonus. Lightly caffeinated green tea gives a gentle lift plus cancer-fighting flavonoids; raw agave sweetens the deal.

1 cup freshly steeped green tea
Juice of 1 medium orange,
    peeled
1 inch fresh gingerroot, peeled
1 tablespoon raw agave
A few drops of liquid
    echinacea
A few drops of liquid zinc

Brew a cup of green tea and add the juiced orange and gingerroot. Stir in the agave, echinacea, and liquid zinc.

Lemon Lozenge

Apple, lemon, and ginger are an immunity boosting power trio, flooding an ailing body with vitamins A, B, and C—plus antioxidants with liver cleansing properties and circulation enhancers. A sprinkle of cayenne helps to relieve congestion and reduce fever.

3 medium apples
½ medium lemon, peeled
1 inch fresh gingerroot, peeled
1 tablespoon raw agave
Pinch of cayenne pepper

Juice the apples, lemon, and gingerroot. Stir together and heat on stove top or using an espresso steamer. Sweeten with the agave and sprinkle with the cayenne pepper.

Ginger Fix

Creamy, spicy, and sweet—this healing tonic is as tasty and restorative as a cup of chai tea. Cinnamon is a powerful antiviral compound also used for its deeply warming properties; practitioners of traditional Chinese medicine often prescribe it to ward off colds. Cardamom is used to treat bronchitis and heal sore throats, and a double dose of ginger works to soothe upper respiratory tract infections and calm nagging coughs.

1 cup almond milk
Juice of 2 inches fresh
    gingerroot, peeled
1 tablespoon raw agave
Pinch of cinnamon
Pinch of cardamom

Stir together and heat on stove top or use an espresso steamer.

Dr. Bombay

Like the best holiday cider boosted with additional beneficial support, this hot blend will calm and comfort on cold and windy days.

Juice of 2½ medium apples
Juice of ½ medium pear
Pinch of cinnamon
A few drops of liquid
    echinacea
A few drops of liquid
    vitamin C
A few drops of liquid zinc

Stir ingredients together and heat on stove top or use an espresso steamer.

JUICY TIP

Liquid forms of the herb echinacea, as well as vitamin C and zinc, can be sourced at health food stores.

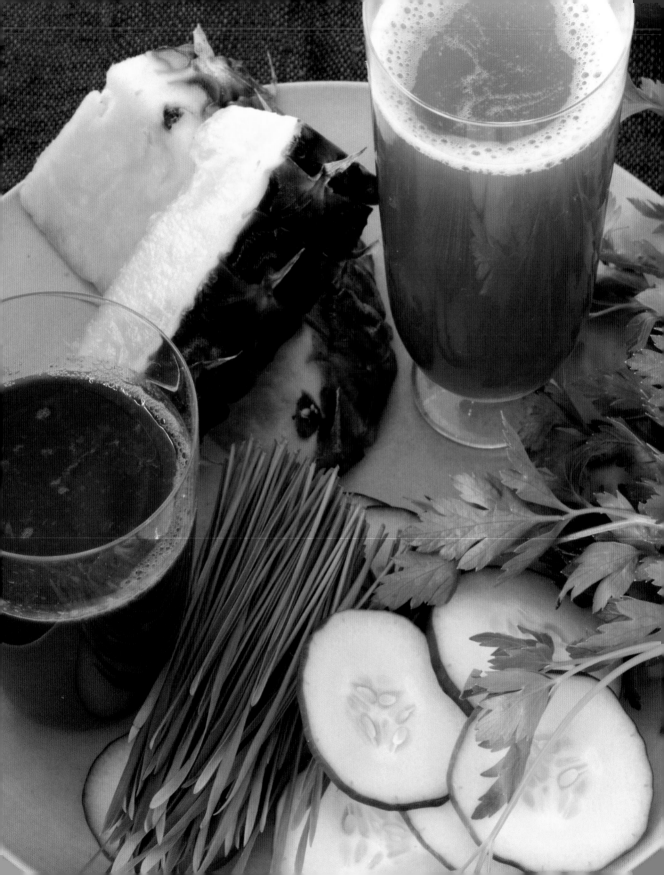

WHEATGRASS RX

The new grass that germinates from wheatberry seeds is considered one of the ultimate "living foods" for its medicinal properties.

Wheatgrass juice became a buzzword in the 70s through its use in progressive healing programs, but now it's embraced by everyday juicers who add it to their diet to maintain optimal health and wellness. Wheatgrass juice helps give a boost to red blood cells, is a powerful detoxifier and alkalinizer, and is so rich in chlorophyll it's sometimes dubbed a liquid oxygen transfusion. Wheatgrass also helps to neutralize environmental toxins in the body and its devotees say it slows the aging process—like a green elixir of youth!

Its strong, grassy taste makes wheatgrass an "advanced green" drink, but mixed into the right juice combo it will be successfully balanced by other flavors. Wheatgrass oxidizes very quickly after juicing and is meant to be consumed right away. Drink the shots or any juice incorporating wheatgrass fresh, rather than storing it in the fridge.

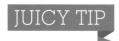

A single or double shot of wheatgrass can be tossed back on its own. Consider it the jade-colored opposite of a steaming espresso shot.

JUICING WHEATGRASS

This delicate plant needs some special care; centrifugal juicers are usually too fast and strong to extract its juice. Masticating juicers usually handle it well, and special wheatgrass juicers are even available. The best way to use it is to purchase large flats of wheatgrass from health food stores or farmers' markets and cut the amount you want to juice each day; some careful tending is required to avoid mold growth at the roots. It's also available precut in bags and should last for up to a week in the fridge. If you fall for the wheatgrass habit, it's relatively simple to grow your own, though your indoor garden will require some daily TLC. Supplies and instructions are easily sourced online.

JUICING JARGON

Chlorophyll is the part of the plant that makes it green. When we consume green plants full of chlorophyll, it has an oxygenating, alkalizing, and purifying effect on our red blood cells and helps to replenish and rebuild them. Chlorophyll also helps to pull out heavy metals from our system, encourages better bowel movements, and promotes good gut flora. It's found in greatest quantity in darker green vegetables like kale, spinach, chard, and arugula; in herbs like parsley and cilantro; in sprouts, and in blue-green algae like chlorella and spirulina, and there's lots of it in wheatgrass. Cooking changes the structure of chlorophyll, which is why juice devotes consider raw juice the most efficient way to get it.

Verdant Vista

The bold green flavor of wheat-grass mingles seamlessly with the fresh sweetness of pineapple and pear—uplifted by a hint of mint—turning this detox drink into a delicious refresher.

2 cups pineapple
½ medium pear
1 sprig mint
Juice.

Top with 1 ounce of wheatgrass juice.

Gaia's Garden

Wheatgrass meets its match with a handful of sweet roots, fortifying leaves, and the refreshing, balancing flavor of cucumber and celery. It's never been so easy to get your grass on.

1 cup spinach
½ medium beet
4 medium carrots
¼ medium cucumber
3 stalks celery
Juice.

Top with 1 ounce of wheatgrass juice.

The Professional

You leave the fruity green drinks to juicing amateurs. You're serious about your greens—and your grass—and your drink shows it. But at Juice Generation, we know that even hardcore green juicers appreciate the lift of a bit of apple and lemon: They turn a good-for-you drink into a tastes-good drink.

2 leaves Swiss chard
1 cup kale
½ cup parsley
3 medium green apples
¼ medium cucumber
½ medium lime, peeled
Juice.

Top with 1 ounce of wheatgrass juice.

JUICE SHOTS

Lots of good things come in a shot glass, but most of them don't make you feel especially great the next day. Juice shots are designed to boost your body when you need a quick hit of high-octane assistance by delivering small but potent doses of curative natural ingredients. Consider them your secret weapons in staying well and vibrant and toss one back the next time you want to rev up your health. Each shot is approximately 1 ounce of juice.

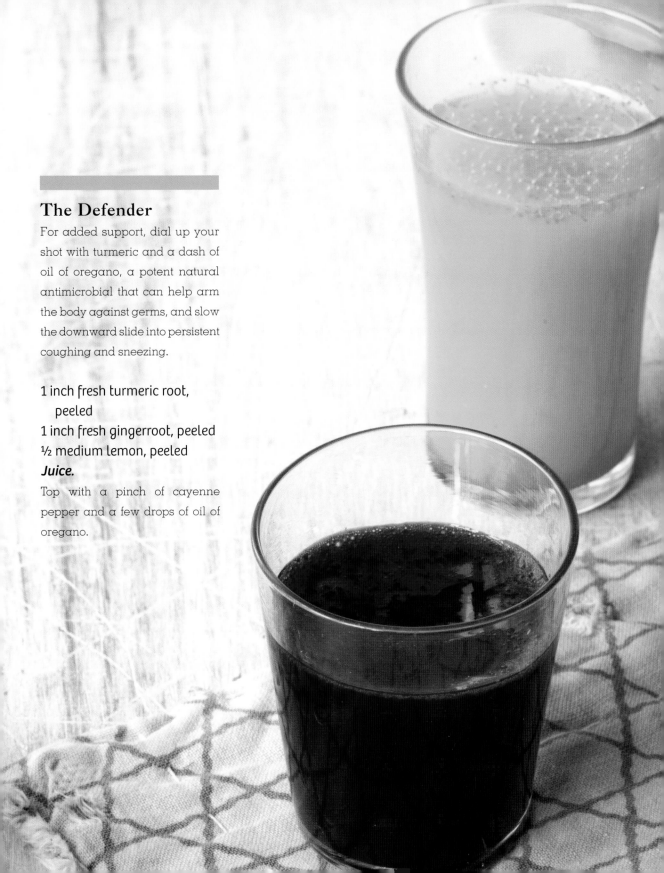

The Defender

For added support, dial up your shot with turmeric and a dash of oil of oregano, a potent natural antimicrobial that can help arm the body against germs, and slow the downward slide into persistent coughing and sneezing.

1 inch fresh turmeric root, peeled
1 inch fresh gingerroot, peeled
½ medium lemon, peeled
Juice.
Top with a pinch of cayenne pepper and a few drops of oil of oregano.

Performance +

At the 2012 London Olympics, word got out that endurance runners and cyclists got juiced on a powerful—and all-natural—performance aid: freshly liquefied beets. The high volume of nitrates in the juice is said to help muscles use oxygen more efficiently, with less fatigue. Not a marathoner? A shot of beet juice delivers the vegetable's liver-boosting and detoxifying properties—without the sugar spike and potential stomach upset of an entire glass. No wonder some natural healers say, "A beet a day keeps the doctor away."

¼ medium beet
½ medium lemon, peeled
Juice.

Fountain of Youth

Legends have been spun around the youth-preserving qualities of bee pollen's tiny golden nuggets. Athletes say the rapidly absorbed, concentrated B vitamins improve strength, endurance, speed, and exercise recovery, while go-go-go urbanites use the "Bs," along with the nuggets' antimicrobial, antibacterial properties, to manage stress and even enhance memory! Bee pollen—the mineral matter gathered by bees as they pollinate plants—is a precious food containing all 22 essential amino acids and the ever-important vitamin B9 (aka folate).

¼ teaspoon bee pollen
1 ounce fresh coconut water
Soak the bee pollen in the coconut water and strain before drinking.

Shot of Gold

While India's ayurvedic doctors consider turmeric a mainstay of health and longevity, protecting the immune system against the effects of stress, India's women know the spice to be a beauty booster, promoting radiant, youthful skin from within. (And without: The powder is often used in rejuvenating face masks.) A shot of juice from the freshly cut root is a whole-food version of the (turmeric-derived) curcumin supplements that are now widely used for wellness. Consider it a daily tonic for body and beauty.

1 inch fresh turmeric root, peeled
½ medium lemon, peeled
Juice.

Vital Shot

At the first sign of a cold, try this warming and cleansing blend of spices, lemon, and healing ginger, to help to fire up your immunity to all-systems-go.

1 inch fresh gingerroot, peeled
½ medium lemon, peeled
Juice.
Top with a pinch of cayenne pepper.

JUICY TIP

Bee pollen can be purchased dried or fresh—the latter has a fluffier texture. Look for raw and unprocessed pollen sourced from your home country. (If the seller does not say where it is from, nix it—it may come from an industrial source and contain contaminants.) Keep it in the fridge, or freezer, to prolong shelf life. It can also boost a smoothie; start with a small amount, such as ¼ teaspoon, gradually working up to more over time (up to 1 tablespoon per drink) if you desire.

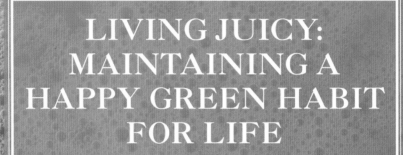

LIVING JUICY: MAINTAINING A HAPPY GREEN HABIT FOR LIFE

THE JUICE GENERATION MANIFESTO

Juicing and blending is for everybody. We believe everybody benefits from an amplification of fresh, uncooked vegetables in their diets, whether it's by a factor of five or fifty, and whatever their diet and lifestyle may be.

Juicing is about more, not less. Enrich your well-being with broad-spectrum nutrition containing a riot of colors and flavors and fun. Juicing is not about denial or stripping anything out of your life.

Simplicity trumps luxury. It does not have to be complicated or lavish to be good for you. What counts is that your juice or blended is made fresh, not bought in packaged, processed versions; that it's made from the best ingredients you can find easily; and that it is balanced in its composition.

Juicing can work your way. There's no need to go extreme or change your whole diet. Learn what type of liquid foods work for you, and ease slowly into your habit. This is concentrated nutrition: A little can go a long way.

Juicing and blending can be a refreshing ritual. Getting your bare hands on piles of fresh and vibrant produce is a ritual that balances the mind, calms the senses, and restores the spirit.

Greens are great health insurance. Don't ditch your regular insurance, but incorporate liquid greens into your diet, and you might not have to claim on it.

A happy green habit that lasts for a lifetime means making juicing and blending work for you. We hope this journey through the three stages of the Green Curve has opened the door to the possibilities of a basket of produce and a pantry of whole foods—and piqued your interest in discovering more from here on out.

Moving forward, use any recipe in this book that you like. Keep a commitment to bring greens and other vibrant colored vegetables into your daily diet, and find the rhythm of juicing or blending that works for you. It may mean making something ultrasimple from Phase 1 with only two or three ingredients; or mixing it up like a master and trying something more complex from Phase 3. Perhaps you'll try adding a new healing ingredient that you sense might help you when you need extra support. And occasionally, you'll try a gentle reset of a liquid-only day (or three). The more you juice and blend, the more you will be able to tune into what your body wants in every moment, and the easier the choices of what to make, and when, will become.

As you continue to purchase produce seasonally and from different vendors, inspiration will probably hit as unexpected vegetables and fruits, along with newly discovered seeds, nuts, and superfoods, fall into your bag. Experiment and enjoy—and remember to share what works!

With your newfound passion for squeezing, crushing, and grinding, you are now an official member of the juice generation. May you always see the wonder in a cucumber, a bunch of spinach, and a handful of berries; may your body always feel the uplifting benefits; and may your curiosity never stop leading you in ever-more-juicy new directions.

ABOUT THE AUTHOR

Eric Helms is the founder of Juice Generation, New York City's premier juicery. Since 1999, his mission has been to create a friendly, accessible juice bar where New Yorkers of all lifestyles could experience the energizing effects of fresh, raw juices. He cofounded the national juice and raw food delivery service, Cooler Cleanse, with Salma Hayek in 2009. He resides in New York City. To learn more about Juice Generation, visit juicegeneration.com.

Amely Greeven is a bestselling writer whose topics include preventive health care, mind-body balance, and the search for peace in modern life. She lives in Southern California and Jackson Hole, Wyoming.

ACKNOWLEDGMENTS

Project Manager
Nazli Kfoury

Creative Director
Marc Balet

Still Life Photography
William Brinson

Lifestyle Photography
John Huba

Design
Tyler Mintz
Cristina Vasquez
Obando

Touchstone
Matthew Benjamin
Stacy Creamer

Juice Generation
Isain Carino
Luis Garcia
Joel Hernandez
Maria Montanez
Emily Parr

Jamie Pelino
Simone Shepard

Special Thanks To
Jake Benson
Whitney Benson
Elyse Connolly
Denise Fiallo
Andrew Ginsburg
Lynn Helms
Jeff Kleinman
Barry Mandel
Shauna Robertson
Jose Tamez
Neal Tully